Organization of Health Workers and Labor Conflict

Edited by Samuel Wolfe

POLICY, POLITICS, HEALTH AND MEDICINE

Series

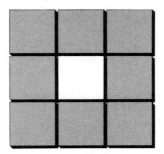

Baywood Publishing Company, Inc.
Farmingdale, New York 11735

Library of Congress Catalog Card Number: 77-94410
ISBN Number: 0-89503-009-8

© 1978, Baywood Publishing Company, Inc.

Library of Congress Cataloging in Publication Data

lectures. I. Wolfe, Samuel. II. International
journal of health services. III. Series.
RA971.35.073   331.88'11'3621   77-94410
ISBN 0-89503-009-8

Main entry under title:

Organization of health workers and labor conflict.

    (Policy, politics, health, and medicine series)
    "Papers ... originally published in the
International journal of health services."
    Includes bibliographical references.
    1. Trade-unions--Health facilities--Addresses,
essays, lectures. 2. Trade-unions--Hospitals--
United States--Addresses, essays, lectures.
3. Social conflict--Addresses, essays, lectures.
4. Nursing--United States--Addresses, essays,
lectures. 5. Women in medicine--Addresses, essays,   __

PREFACE

The papers presented in this collection, originally published in the *International Journal of Health Services,* represent various points of view relating to the organization of health workers and to labor conflict in the health sector. While these papers are by no means all inclusive of the field, they include selections from writers concerning the United States and four other widely different countries.

Part 1, titled *Worker Conflict in the Health Field* includes eight papers about the United States, Canada, Chile, and Great Britain. What seems to emerge are differing ways to handle conflicts with more professionalized workers on the one hand, and on the other hand with semi skilled and relatively unskilled health workers. From the United States come the voices of hospital management, of the health and hospital workers, and of an organizer of physicians into unions. From Canada, Robin Badgley, and from the United States, Barbara and John Ehrenreich, discuss the social and economic basis for labor conflict in the health sector, and the underlying class conflicts and conflicts over societal inequality that relate to the conflicts. Belmar and Sidel describe poignantly the doctors' strikes in Chile, and the role these played in the overthrow of the elected government of Chile and the murder of its physician-President. Widgery underscores the unrest in Britain, relating to both medical care and political issues, that have led to labor unrest in the health field in that country.

Part 2, titled *Allied Workers, Nurses, Women* contains five chapters. The first, by Carol Brown, focuses on the expansion of allied health work and the mechanisms maintained by the medical profession to retain a virtual total control over these expanding occupations. Cannings and Lazonick trace the development of the nursing labor force in the United States, the trend to worker organization in this huge labor force, and the potential for an organized nursing labor force to give leadership in restructuring the health services in the United States. In another selection by Carol Brown, she analyzes the predominant number of women health workers—and the predominant control over them by men. Occupation, woman-woman, and man-woman conflicts are frequent, and such conflicts must be overcome if women are to succeed in organizing, in unionizing, in order to change the status of women in the health field. Bonnie Bullough spells out the barriers to the nurse practitioner movement: the traditional subordinate role of women (nurses) to men (physicians) in our society is again played out in the nurse practitioner-physician "games," and such patterns are barriers that prevent the full flowering of nurses as practitioners. In the final paper, Magdalena Sokolowska, the distinguished Polish physician-sociologist, takes a more general look at the determinants of occupational position among all women workers in Poland: again one finds continued disparities based on sexual discrimination.

Taken together, these papers represent—not a unified theme and a coherent whole—but an introduction to factors associated with health worker organization, labor conflict and the underlying class and class-related sex and ethnic conflicts that beset the health sector in various countries. That these conflicts will not go away is clear. How to channel them into constructive struggle for social and societal change is the dilemma to be faced.

Samuel Wolfe
Columbia University

Acknowledgement—Thanks are extended to Hila Richardson for her help in selecting the papers for this volume. Special thanks to Vicente Navarro, of Johns Hopkins University, for his role in founding the *International Journal of Health Services,* which has become an important vehicle for exchange on topics such as those presented in this volume.

TABLE OF CONTENTS

PART 1

Worker Conflict in the Health Field

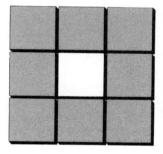

CHAPTER 1

Worker Conflicts In The Health Field: An Overview

Samuel Wolfe

In addition to this overview, seven papers on the theme of worker conflicts in the health field are presented in this part of the volume. These interesting and probably controversial papers present a wide spectrum of information, as well as a substantial range of ideological views. These papers taken together show us what nonsense it is to believe, as some have said, that we are at the end of ideology. What these papers tell us, in my view, is that the world as we know it is in the midst of frightening but exhilarating conflicts and upheavals, and these conflicts in the health sector are in microcosm a reflection of the tensions of the larger world of which health care is but a small part.

Robin Badgley of Canada has written on the social and economic bases of conflict among health workers. Stressing the alienation of people from their work and the status inconsistencies and relative economic deprivation of whole groupings of health workers, he shows that the trend toward unionization and conflict and strikes has been inevitable. Badgley concludes that if the rights and health of patients and public can be preserved, then strikes can be an important catalyst for change in a society such as ours. Strikes highlight the need for structural change in redefining the needs of workers, especially of lower- and middle-echelon workers. Yet, unionization of health workers and the pressures toward more stringent cost controls in the health field clash head on; with jobs being reclassified and redefined as a result, and with necessary preoccupation with cost efficiency, increasing conflicts may be anticipated in the years ahead.

Davis and Foner, trade union leaders who have played key roles in organizing low-income health workers, point out that the vast majority of such workers are not organized. They remind us that many of these workers are women, poor, black, and Spanish-speaking, and are traditionally exploited by the larger society. They describe the benefits of unionization and the broader social goals of the union, which have included important links with the United States civil rights movement.

Match, Goldstein, and Light, in expressing the position of hospital management, point out that hospitals are increasingly in a bind. They have fixed numbers of dollars and growing pressures for the use of these fixed dollars. Increasingly, the hospital is really the middle man in negotiations since in order to increase their revenues, hospitals have to get approval from state agencies, which in turn leads to higher premium rates for the insured population. These authors, intensely unhappy about strike action by hospital workers, propose binding arbitration by outside arbitrators who do not have local vested interests when they enter into participation in a dispute.

Sanford Marcus, a physician engaged in organizing physicians into trade unions, feels that the inexorable forces of the insurance industry, the hospital industry, and government involvement in the financing of health care have led to medical unionism. Thereby, says Marcus, doctors can best protect their own interests and by so doing they can also serve as effective consumer advocates.

Barbara and John Ehrenreich note that hospital workers, like other workers, need meaningful work and adequate recognition in terms of money, respect, and status. These needs are frustrated by the conditions of work in the large modern hospital—for the unskilled and the semiskilled there are forces that lead to the typical industrial work ethic and alienation from the content of work. For the skilled, there is the ideology of professionalism. Clear-cut class conflicts are in the making based on divisions with opposing class identifications: on the one hand a proletarianized body of unskilled and semiskilled workers, and on the other, a large group of skilled workers who are allowed, through their professionalism, to participate in the real status of doctors.

Roberto Belmar, formerly of Chile, and Victor Sidel of New York have written a moving account of the background to the doctors' strikes in Chile. The medical profession was opposed to government programs for community participation in health and for changes in the models for delivery of health care, and feared a change in the status of physicians. But there were also broader links between the organized medical profession and the political opponents of the government of Dr. Salvador Allende, the socialist physician who had been democratically elected as the president of Chile. Thus, the medical profession played an active role in the overthrow of the government and in the murder of Dr. Allende and many of his supporters.

David Widgery of Great Britain traces the background and development of the main manual and white-collar trade unions in health care in Great Britain, before and after the creation of the National Health Service in 1948, and the wave of actions including strikes in British hospitals over the past several years. These strikes, while seen as a last resort tactic by manual workers pressing for more wages, have actually been part of more widespread actions by all types of hospital workers, have ranged over various political and health care issues, and have played a key role in the debate over the future of the British National Health Service.

While Drs. Belmar and Sidel may not agree with me, in my judgment there were striking similarities between the behavior of the medical profession in Chile in 1972 - 1973 and the behavior of the medical profession before and during the doctors' strike in Saskatchewan, Canada, in 1962 (1). At that time, the democratically elected social democrat government of that province of Canada had decided to implement a plan, compulsory in nature, to pay all doctors' bills, and had been reelected to power with a mandate to do so. Pressure groups, including the medical profession, abused the democratic process. A coalition consisting of the medical profession, the business community, chambers of commerce, and other professions representing wealth and power groupings in our society, attempted to subvert the legislation to which a duly elected government had been committed. That was the overriding issue at the time. These same forces led a campaign which defeated the government at the polls in the 1964 election.

In a subsequent essay, Badgley and I discussed the question of the doctors' right to strike (2). A recent review of that essay suggests that the position we took in 1968 may still be relevant in the mid 1970s. We pointed out that in the next generation the great majority of physicians will find themselves in bureaucratic organizations. Such physicians ought to have the right to negotiate. Increasingly, their goals will be more like those of other trade unionists. Yet the majority of the medical profession still denies the public the right to negotiate the price of physician services. Increasingly, such prices, and arrangements for payment for physician services, will come to be negotiated rather than unilaterally imposed, even in the United States. Under such circumstances, greater conflicts are bound to arise. While compromises and concessions are necessary in such conflicts, the line must be drawn—it is an illegal and criminal act for a physician to withdraw his services from the sick, or to abandon his patients. Thus, there is a need to assure satisfactory negotiating mechanisms.

How can this be done? There is no sure way. There should be built in and clearly spelled out mechanisms for mediation, for conciliation, and for the use of prestigious fact-finding tribunals; these are necessary preliminaries to the submission to binding arbitration of unresolved differences.

For physicians, as for other workers, unless the arbitration results in an award that is grossly unjust, patently absurd, or technically defective, then there ought to be the assumption that the agreement is binding and acceptable to both sides. And while ideally an individual doctor should be able to opt out of a contract with a third party—and this is an important civil right for a doctor—opting out on a large scale as a strategy to circumvent negotiations and arbitration would be a clear demonstration of bad faith. Thus, physicians in countries such as Canada and the United States—at least for the next decade or two—ought to be in bargaining units, and the units should represent those who are in them; if the majority accepts a contract, then surely it will be binding on all those covered by the contract. And it follows that while the medical profession can withdraw its services from a contract with government or with the other third parties, it cannot withdraw its services from the public.[1]

Badgley points out in his paper that when health workers have gone on strike in Canada, penalties have been inversely imposed by the courts depending on the status of the occupations involved: no sanctions have been used against striking doctors, while other striking health workers have been threatened with fines, firing, or prison sentences.

The strike by Local 1199 against hospitals in the metropolitan New York area in late 1973 is a classic example of class conflict. These low-income strikers, by and large semiskilled and unskilled, and by and large black or Hispanic, and their union leaders, were the objects of ridicule of the boards of directors and medical staffs of the affected hospitals. And in truth, some strikers did act badly. Patient care may have been affected. But within the hospitals, there was joyousness amidst tension. For the doctors and those social workers and other health professionals who were not in the union, and the members of the boards of directors, for a few days did the work of the people standing on the picket lines: cook food, feed patients, clean toilets, scrub floors, do typing, take messages, and so on and so on. These persons, who on the average earned from 4 to 15 times as much as did the workers on the picket lines, felt cleansed by their participation in menial tasks for this brief period of time. Not only were they providing a useful service but at the same time they could feel righteously or self-righteously indignant at those who had walked off their jobs.

Yet the key high-income actors in this little drama would be horrified if *they* were accused of having been *on strike* over the years. For the hospital boards of directors—weren't they over the years really standing apart from many of the critical needs of the community they were supposed to serve? And who really sat on the board? How many ordinary workers? How many trade unionists? And how many lawyers, real

---

[1] Badgley and I, during our earlier work on this subject, were helped very much by the thinking of the late Andrew Andras, who at the time was Director of Legislation, Canadian Labour Congress, Ottawa.

estate speculators, bankers, and well-to-do businessmen? And if philanthropy contributes less than 1 per cent of hospital operating budgets, why are 75 to 95 per cent of the boards made up of those who are rich?

And if the hospital is serious about its business and its responsiblity, why is it that the emergency rooms and outpatient clinics—where many low-income workers and their families get their usual care—have such poor services? Why are the affluent doctors not working regularly in these settings, where the need is so great? Why are they often allowed incomes of up to $100,000 per year (if one includes fringe benefits) plus additional income from their private practices *within* these same hospitals, by these same boards of directors, and yet allowed to walk away from accepting responsibility for the chaos that is the ambulatory services in most hospitals in America?

These questions are not meant to divide people. These are the observable realities which, as the Ehrenreichs and Badgley have stressed in the papers that follow, give rise to the class conflicts that are coming to the fore in the health sector. Given the present arrangements for organization and financing of health services, and the way in which power is structured and controlled in the health services (of which the complex hospital is a prototype), there is every reason to believe that the have-nots of our society, the traditional menials of the health care system, will become better organized to demand a narrowing of the gap between their income and status and those of the haves in the health system. After all, if altruism has become a rare commodity among physician-healers, why should it be a common commodity in the ward aide or the janitor at the hospital?

The struggle for union recognition and the associated right to strike by relatively low-income workers has entirely different origins than do similar efforts by highly professionalized health workers such as physicians. In the one case, the attempt is being made to change the status quo or at least to widen the cast of players who participate in the status quo, and in the other, to maintain things as they are. In the one case, the relative irreplaceability, for certain tasks, of the scarce skills of physicians confers such power on them that society has the duty to restrict the total right to independent actions; thus, the right to collective withdrawal of services, such as through strike action, has to be denied. But such a right, clearly, ought *not* to be denied to the lower- and middle-echelon workers, who have organized themselves for collective action, since, as has been indicated above, such persons are replaceable and dispensable; for most of their everyday tasks, the physician, lawyer or housewife can step into the breach and act as substitutes for them in their work. This vulnerability to being readily replaced should, in a society such as ours, give them the right to strike.

Therein lies the source of future class conflict in the larger society, and assuredly, in the health sector. We have, as Jeremy Brecher (3) points out in an excellent recent book on strikes, been dominated by the consensus school, as though it was benign, when in fact there is good evidence that threat has been a constant factor in moulding the so-called American Consensus; repression is absent only when the status quo is unchallenged. Class conflict has always been a reality in our society. Now let us begin to talk about it more, and perhaps to do something about it.

REFERENCES

1. Badgley, R. F., and Wolfe, S. *Doctors' Strike. Medical Care and Conflict in Saskatchewan.* Macmillan of Canada, Toronto, 1967 and 1971.
2. Badgley, R. F., and Wolfe, S. The doctors' right to strike. In *Ethical Issues in Medicine*, edited by E. F. Torrey, Ch. 15. Little, Brown, Boston, 1968.
3. Brecher, J. *Strike!* (The True History of Mass Insurgence in America from 1877 to the Present—as authentic revolutionary movements against the establishments of state, capital and trade unionism.) Straight Arrow Books, San Francisco, 1972.

CHAPTER 2

Health Worker Strikes:
Social And Economic
Bases Of Conflict

Robin F. Badgley

In few other institutions of society is social and economic inequality among workers so marked and yet so generally unacknowledged as in the health systems of the western nations. The enclosed structure of health occupations in the 20th century retains attributes reminiscent of a feudal society, in which there is rigid persistence of privileged job titles, distinctive and symbolic work attire, apprenticeship training, guild-like professional associations, preferential codes of ethics and, above all, a rigid and an unequal system of economic and social rewards among workers.

Under state health insurance or social security programs—measures intended for the public good—workers at the top of the hierarchy have gained in income and social prestige while middle and lower echelon workers have suffered regressive consequences of the programs, resulting in a growing mood of dissatisfaction and a feeling of "being left out." Inasmuch as health values represent core social priorities, this inequitable structure of the health system has for the most part remained unchallenged and, until recent years, relatively free of conflict.

The tranquility of the health marketplace is now being jolted by a growing number of strikes, threats of strikes, "booking off," or work-to-rule campaigns by workers ranging from housekeeping staff to physicians. Some recent instances[1] include:

- Sixteen doctors' strikes in seven European countries, 1960-1968;
- Strikes by nurses, hospital workers, and ambulance drivers in the United Kingdom, 1973-1974;
- Strikes by New York City hospital workers (1973) and California nurses (1974);
- A 48-hour all health workers' strike against the policies of the late Chilean President Salvador Allende (1973);
- A two-day strike by Italian physicians (1974);
- Approximately 40 strikes or threatened strikes by all categories of health workers in Canada since 1970.

Despite the apparently growing number of disputes in health labor relations, the predominant emphasis in discussions of health affairs has been on the distribution of

---

[1] The trends listed here are incomplete, being derived from reports in professional journals and newspapers. In Canada, strikes and (in parentheses) threatened strikes from 1972 to 1974 included: physicians and interns, 0 (3); nurses, 4 (5); technical personnel, 3 (3); nonmedical workers, 12 (2); federal and provincial public health workers, 1 (3); and nursing home employees, 1 (3).

outcome indices, the portrayal of the health system as a stable institution, or the fostering of consumer participation. These concerns have implicitly diverted attention from questions such as how the internal division of labor in the health system is structured, how it changes, and how conflict and its effects are resolved.

A strike is a collective and ultimate step by workers who seek to ameliorate their working conditions—in essence, to alter specified conditions of the status quo. In some industries strikes have become an accepted, almost endemic way of resolving contract disputes between management and labor. This has not been the case among health workers, where wildcat strikes are rare and where legal injunctions may prohibit the disruption of "essential" community services. Strikes by health workers, usually premeditated collective actions taken with the realization that deeply rooted ethical and perhaps legal principles are being broken, have not yet resolved the underlying institutional seeds of work conflict. Strikes by doctors, for instance, represent broad and fundamental shifts in the nature of job values held by society and in the shape of the health system itself.

ALIENATION AND HEALTH WORK

In a vast bureaucracy, economic power and social status are precious commodities. Workers are often rewarded by how much money they earn as well as by the length of their vacations, the size and decor of their work place, or the nature of other fringe benefits. If these benefits are unequally dispersed, increased for some workers but not for others, or if sharp discrepancies develop between income and perceived status, then discontent, high job turnover, and conflict usually result.

As large bureaucracies expand to encompass previously dispersed or uncoordinated institutions, two counterforces are emerging in many western nations to challenge the established social division of labor among workers. Reacting to the growing concentration of power in large corporations, workers increasingly are joining unions in many industries and are aggressively pressing for higher wages and increased job benefits. The trend toward unionization has been complemented by the socially corrosive effects of monetary inflation, with its invidious wage-price spread consequences for workers with various levels of training or those working in the public versus private sectors of the economy. These combined forces are now uniting many workers whose interests previously had been unarticulated or unorganized. Particularly affected are workers employed by those corporate elements under public authority, for under these circumstances it is difficult for preset tax rates or specified prices for services to keep pace with rising costs.

Many state health insurance programs now face a dilemma: How can they remain within established fiscal guidelines and at the same time accommodate their large corporate structures to meet the current inflation spiral and the demands which are resulting in the growing unionization of health workers? While in some instances these trends may be short-lived, they could leave a durable imprint on the structure of health labor relations. The experience of one nation, Canada, provides an example of management-labor trends in health services which may be occurring in other western nations. In Canada, the impact of large state-run health corporations, growing unionization among workers, and wage discrepancies triggered by monetary inflation is resulting in increased labor unrest and strikes by health workers. The general consequences of these changes are (a) gradual erosion of professional autonomy; (b) emergence of social pressures stemming from job status inconsistencies; and (c) increased importance of relative income levels.

Professional Autonomy

Health professions have traditionally prided themselves on governing their own affairs, an authority confirmed by the state. This power of the major professions has spread like a web to control training schools, hospital operations, and tariff schedules, and to constrain competitor disciplines. These customs have become so entrenched that professional leaders in some nations hold them to be inviolable rights which, if altered, would reduce the quality of their services provided to the public.

Legislators who monitor expenditures from the public sector are increasingly seeking to establish a balance between competing social priorities, meet the health needs voiced by the public, and still provide health services more economically. As the state through its health service corporate elements introduces controls by limiting the expansion of hospitals, by decisions on the channeling of research monies, or by negotiating wage increases, health professionals in many western nations have predictably opposed this erosion of their established powers. When the issues fail to reach a point of open conflict and instead simmer with broad-felt discontent, one option sometimes taken by highly trained health professionals is to emigrate to nations where it is felt that the freedom of professional autonomy is still preserved. However, it should be noted that this autonomy is under assault even in the United States, the country to which many have emigrated.

Once health insurance measures have been introduced, such programs have usually not remained static for long. Canada, for instance, introduced its national medicare program in 1968. Since that time steps taken by some provinces to limit professional powers have included, inter alia: the imposition of income ceilings; the revision of professional codes; auditing by the state of professional practice; lay participation on disciplinary boards; mandatory postgraduate study to retain state licensing prerogatives; provincial quotas imposed on medical schools in the graduation of family doctors; limiting of residency training programs; and setting of regional quotas on hospital beds.

The medical profession in Canada has twice gone on strike (in Saskatchewan and in Quebec) and on several other occasions has threatened to boycott health measures introduced by government (1-6). In each instance the question of who governs for the public good was a central issue in the test of professional versus state power. The results of the last two doctors' strikes (in 1962 and 1970) made the medical profession throughout Canada more willing to negotiate with the state over a number of issues which it previously considered solely within its domain. Gone are the days when a Canadian medical leader could assert: "What is best for the medical profession must be best for the public" (7). The strategy for the control of major health professions of various provincial governments in Canada has involved the commissioning of task force reports and usually extensive prior consultation with medical leaders, steps which have typically led to the introduction of compromise measures. Although both sides seem to win in this process, the direction and tempo of events favor the state and the power of the professions in Canada is slowly eroded. The introduction of these controls has been softened by the fact that physicians' incomes have been allowed to soar above pre-state-health-insurance levels. Physicians thus seem to enjoy a high degree of autonomy but in reality are more accountable to the state than ever before. Potential conflict in this instance has been avoided by a strategy of gradual accommodation, a process whereby issues which were only vaguely defined by the state have been sharply defined by doctors' strikes or incipient conflict.

At least in Canada, and, it would seem, elsewhere as well, major associations of professional health workers are beginning to resemble labor unions. As one former provincial medical association president put it: "Only the development of medical trade unions with a hard-headed willingness to disrupt society . . . will roll back this obstruction in communication between our political masters and those who . . . provide health care" (8). The professions negotiate contracts with management, in this case the state. There is an open acknowledgment of concern with wages, working conditions, and fringe job benefits. As organized medicine takes on these attributes or as doctors' unions emerge, a new sense of militancy is replacing the previous stance before the public of professional aloofness concerning pecuniary issues. The change is of benefit to the public: there is more direct social responsibility than before on the part of these occupations essential to the public well-being. No longer do leaders unilaterally set the terms of reference for the profession, and no longer are they held to be above the social controls imposed by the state on its workers.

Status Inconsistency

Sharp job and personal status inconsistencies have been tolerated as integral dimensions of middle-level health service work. While purporting to be self-governing professions, these occupations have exercised only partial work autonomy, have received relatively low wages, and have been required to maintain personally disruptive work schedules. A division of labor by sex has often reinforced the subordinate vocational status of these jobs by social definitions of what constitutes appropriate work for women. Partly for these reasons and also because of the quasi-military history of some of these fields of endeavor, status symbolism has been stressed in lieu of remuneration or job benefits. For example, few other occupations have taken so much pride as nursing in the accoutrements of occupational attire and yet at the same time have been so easily co-opted by the conservative attitudes toward labor relations often held by health administrators.

The social composition of this middle-level work force, with its short-term career commitment and high job turnover rates, has limited the growth of strong associations or constrained a sense of militancy from developing among workers about their working conditions. If staff supervision or work conditions were unsatisfactory, the easiest choice was to move to another setting. Hospital and health administrators have rationalized these trends as stemming from the lack of career aspirations of young women and have done little to modify existing work routines or to provide socially satisfactory career lines.

This acquiescent mood is now changing as some middle-level health workers see their income equaled or exceeded by workers with less formal training whom they reject as their status equals. The slow build-up of job frustration has also been fueled by a fresh awareness of women's rights, by the impact of inflation, and by disenchantment with traditional prestige symbols. This stance has been well caught in placards used by nurses picketing a provincial legislature in Canada:

> Florence had a little lamp
> She carried it with pride;
> But when she saw her paycheck
> Even she sat down and cried.

Unionization, previously an anathema to middle-level health workers, is now transforming existing associations or leading to the formation of new, more adamant groups which are challenging all aspects of the status quo. Since 1970, in Canada, there have been approximately 40 strikes or threatened strikes by hospital and public health nurses, laboratory technicians, or Indian medical services personnel. No national associations have developed to press the interests of these workers, but the residue of militancy generated has altered negotiations throughout the country. More universalistic national job norms are developing, with the result that regional disparities are being reduced in the wage settlements which are reached.

These changes represent a growing sense of job alienation. Middle-level workers, formerly affiliated with local hospitals or training centers, are now under the direction of a diffuse, often unknown regional center where decisions are made about personnel quotas, training curricula, and uniform job specifications. Thus while health systems are becoming more rational and, in terms of benefits for the public, possibly more equitable, the overall effect has been an increase in the level of voiced dissatisfaction among these workers, and in turn an accelerated growth of health service unions.

Relative Deprivation

Studies of health services by government commissions or scholars have generally been preoccupied with high-level workers such as doctors, dentists, or nurses. In Canada in the past decade, for instance, there have been a dozen major provincial or federal reviews of health manpower trends, but no study has dealt in depth with the job requirements or work problems of lower-level nonmedical workers. A growing sense of dissatisfaction among these workers in some instances has resulted from a widening gap between their incomes and those of other health jobs or, in many settings, with similar work done for private enterprise. The working conditions of these forgotten men and women who do the menial work in the health services sector have remained relatively unchanged for years. In comparison with other workers they are often underpaid, they have been poorly organized, and they have been ignored by strong industrial unions and upper-echelon health officials.

Because in the past health care fused religious and philanthropic values of personal service, it became customary to provide low wages and minimal fringe benefits for nursing assistants, orderlies, maintenance personnel, and the laundry, dietary, and general housekeeping hospital staff. These workers were expected to endorse the altruistic values of the major health professions without receiving their own proportional acknowledgment in the form of income or prestige rewards. This income structure is now being widely challenged by nonmedical workers who seek higher incomes and better working conditions. An anomaly emerges when the work which they do is compared with how society recognizes or recompenses their efforts. As many studies have found, nonmedical and nonnursing hospital staff may have contacts with patients at least as extensive as those of doctors or nurses; their communication makes an effective contribution to the social side of patient care. Yet despite this involvement in patient care they are not paid for these functions and are relegated to the lower rungs of prestige in the health hierarchy.

In Canada, where strikes by health workers are prohibited by law in most provinces, penalties have been inversely imposed by the courts according to the status of the occupations involved. No sanctions have been used against striking doctors. In contrast, some striking nurses or nonmedical workers have been fined or threatened with fines, fired, or given a prison sentence.

This morally untenable situation raises the broader issue of what sanctions society can effectively impose on a prestigious and technically irreplaceable group of workers who go on strike. Were doctors, for instance, to withdraw their services completely for an extended period, the only recourse available to the state to maintain the necessary health care would be to seek emergency medical assistance from other nations. This is not the case when other health workers strike, because their services can be provided at least on an interim basis by physicians or other personnel. The hypothetical total doctors' strike underscores the variable use of sanctions by society in disputes among health workers as well as the powerful bargaining position held by certain major health professions.

In some western nations the position of lower-level health workers is being recognized by organized labor, which in the past found it difficult to organize union locals among service workers.[2] In Canada several national unions are moving in this direction and are providing experienced leadership by drawing upon established union resources. The position taken by union leaders is becoming more adamant, and as one spokesman has asserted: "We are going to have to strike. There are going to be violations of the law. There is no other way out. We are continuing to fall behind workers in outside industries" (9). As this "catch up" trend is established, it may bring the income levels of these jobs in line with wages paid to comparable workers in industry, stiffen the bargaining positions of middle-level workers, and change the nature of the sanctions used against strikes in health services.

POTENTIAL CATALYST FOR CHANGE

National legislatures are one means of controlling the functions and working conditions of complex state health insurance programs. Other checks which modify the dominant command of resources wielded by vast health institutions include competing social priorities, the aims of the concerned professions, and the extent to which workers in the health system concur or dissent with its purposes. In many nations where state health insurance has been enacted, the public regards health care as a social right rather than a privilege bestowed by altruistic personnel, and health workers increasingly emphasize the scope of their job benefits. Although some public leaders reject strikes by health workers as illegal or unethical, "the loss of an essential community service," or "injurious to patients," there is little or no evidence that the health of either individual patients or of the public has been substantially harmed in any instance. Almost invariably, alternate arrangements have been made for the care of chronic patients and emergency services have been established for individuals with acute illnesses.

The strikes which have taken place have usually led to short-term gains rather than to any radical reshaping of the health system. However, radical reshaping has seldom been the objective of striking workers. Because their interests are fragmented by technical divisions of labor and different career aims, they have seldom spoken simultaneously or unanimously. Unions of health workers have as yet been weak, have tended to have inexperienced direction, and have been intimidated in their affairs by the dominant health professions. There are indications in some nations that these circumstances may be changing, and the effects of growing tension and unionization will have far-reaching repercussions in the future.

---

[2] *Editor's Note*—The contribution by Davis and Foner in this issue of the *Journal* is illustrative of this trend.

The trend toward the unionization of health workers leaves many questions unanswered. Under what conditions do strong unions emerge? What has been their impact on reshaping prevailing health policies? Under what conditions do health workers go on strike and with what consequences for the public, themselves, and the health system? What sanctions are used by society against strikes by health workers? How and to whom are these sanctions applied? Despite these and other unresolved issues, *if the rights and health of patients and the public are preserved*, then strikes can serve as an important catalyst in converting a rigid and conservative health system into a more flexible democratic organization for all of its workers. The argument against allowing strikes by health workers—i.e. that innocent people suffer harm—remains unproven. It is more often advanced in order to maintain a system's status quo and preserve an invidious stance in the name of ethics than to deal directly with the conditions causing worker dissatisfaction.

Strikes highlight the need for structural change, particularly in redefining the work needs of middle- and lower-echelon health workers. The opinion of these workers is seldom represented or sought out in various health councils. In this respect civil service health bureaucracies mirror the power structure of the health system with professionally trained policy makers holding the positions of authority and rank-and-file workers being rarely represented. Yet the extent of participation or nonparticipation of lower-echelon workers in these public corporations is by itself a measure of the dynamic and equitable structure of a health system.

In his essay on *Class, Citizenship and Social Development*, T. H. Marshall (10) argues that the extent to which citizenship rights were historically available to a population is a fundamental index of a nation's social ideology. Where these rights have been held by a small social elite, this entrenched concentration of power has fostered revolutionary activities. By analogy, if the health system in many western nations remains rigid and authoritarian under the changing tide of current social forces, sharper conflict than has yet been experienced can be expected in the future.

Social choices other than that of maintaining the current health structure are available even in a western democratic society, but many of these are now regarded by most individuals as unacceptable options, and their possible implementation derives from each nation's priorities. These feasible social options in the health system include:

- An equitable and standardized means of paying all workers in accord with their experience and training;
- A payment formula which includes all health occupational categories;
- The establishment where these do not exist of the rights of workers to collective bargaining;
- Establishing criteria for the selection of arbitrators and for determining wage rates for health personnel;
- The proportional representation by job category in health councils at all levels from hospitals to government advisory boards;
- The functional realignment of established health job functions;
- The facilitating of vocational mobility between health jobs by the interlocking of training programs;
- *With necessary public safeguards* ensured, the legalizing of strikes by health workers.

These changes would foster an internal dynamism in the health system which is now often lacking.

The social intent of unionization and strikes to extend job benefits raises the critical issue of how health is valued and paid for by society as a social priority. If, as a result of worker militancy, wage levels are merely raised without corresponding cutbacks elsewhere in the health system, then the total costs generated to be drawn from the public purse will increase proportionately. To meet sharply rising health costs, many countries are already seeking to limit expenditures by imposing fiscal guidelines. These two countertrends, unionization and cost controls, may thrust the health system on a critical cost-efficiency course in the future, affecting the established functions now performed by most health workers. Some jobs inevitably would be found to be duplicative or redundant. Implicitly, strikes by health workers make the distinction between the provision of necessary, minimal care for patients and the established but not optimal current organization of health services. This fact is underscored by a recent U.S. Navy Technomics study of 50 health occupations (11). Of 18,500 job tasks which were identified, 7,000 were considered essential for good health care, and these could be regrouped functionally into 16 job categories.

The potential 68 per cent reduction in health jobs and the 62 per cent overlap in work functions indicate that much of the structure of the health system is maintained by established vocational interests and customs rather than being derived directly from the nature of the services which need to be done. The fight to index wage scales and develop uniform job specifications is kindling a vigorous spirit of unity among some health workers. However, as Karl Marx observed almost a century ago, the growth of unions demanding higher wages is not synonymous with a movement among workers to change existing work conditions or to restructure a system.

What is now happening in the health affairs of certain western nations is the development of a key premise of Marx, namely, the unionization of health workers who are seeking better wages. However, if this occurs alone, and broader changes in the health system do not take place along the lines of feasible social options, then the prospect is that the emphasis on wages will reinforce under new conditions the current rigid and inflexible structure of the hierarchy in health jobs. If this development occurs, and there are strong indications that it will, then the codifying of job functions sought by unions will make it more difficult to realign work tasks, will thwart efforts to constrain rising health costs, and will leave lower-echelon health workers in a position where they are no better off than they now are in terms of relative income or social status.

The basic issue is not whether controversy in the form of work-to-rule campaigns or strikes in the health systems of western nations will subside or increase, but whether such conflict will be anticipated and structurally channeled to increase the satisfaction of health workers and in turn achieve the target of good health for the public. When and how these purposes are attained is a moral issue for each nation to resolve according to its concern for achieving social equity for those who receive services as well as for those workers at all levels who provide them to the public.

Acknowledgments—For their review of a preliminary draft of this paper, I acknowledge with appreciation the perceptive comments of D. Coburn, M. J. Kelner, P. K-M. New, and G. Torrance.

REFERENCES

1. Cassidy, H. M. *Social Security and Reconstruction in Canada*. Ryerson Press, Toronto, 1943.
2. Cassidy, H. M. *Public Health and Welfare Reorganization*. Ryerson Press, Toronto, 1945.
3. Badgley, R. F., and Wolfe, S. *Doctors' Strike: Medical Care and Conflict in Saskatchewan*. Atherton Press, New York, 1967; Macmillan Company, Toronto, 1967 and 1971.
4. Wolfe, S., and Badgley, R. F. *The Family Doctor*. Macmillan Company, Toronto, 1972.
5. Taylor, M. G. Quebec Medicare: Policy formulation in conflict and crisis. *Canadian Public Administration* 211-250, Summer 1972.
6. Badgley, R. F., and Charles, C. A., with Anderson, O. W. The Canadian experience with universal health insurance, unpublished working report, U.S.–HSM 110-71-278, 1971-1975.
7. A plan for health insurance. *Can. Med. Assoc. J.* September Supplement, p. 26, 1934.
8. *Toronto Star*, p. 42. May 19, 1972.
9. *Toronto Globe and Mail*, p. 1, November 9, 1972.
10. Marshall, T. H. *Class, Citizenship and Social Development*. Doubleday-Anchor, Garden City, N.J., 1965.
11. Cooper, J. A. D. Symposium on career development of health professionals. 139th Meeting of the American Association for the Advancement of Science, Washington, D.C., December 27, 1972.

CHAPTER 3

Organization And Unionization
Of Health Workers
In The United States:
The Trade Union Perspective

Leon J. Davis and Moe Foner

A DOOR OPENS FOR WORKERS

The United States Congress has recently passed legislation removing the exemption of voluntary, or nonprofit, hospitals and nursing homes from coverage under the National Labor Relations Act. The new law, enacted on August 25, 1974, rights an historic injustice by extending collective bargaining rights to the country's 1.5 million employees of voluntary hospitals. This legislation, long a goal of the National Union of Hospital and Health Care Employees, in which District 1199 plays a key role, opens the door to the organization of hospital workers on a nationwide scale. It received the strong support of the AFL-CIO and was bitterly opposed by the American Hospital Association.

LOW LEVEL OF UNIONIZATION AND POOR WAGES OF HEALTH WORKERS

The potential for the organization of voluntary hospital employees is enormous. Of the 1.5 million workers in these institutions fewer than 300,000 belong to unions. The three largest and most active unions in the health field today are 1199's National Union of Hospital and Health Care Employees, the Service Employees International Union (SEIU), and the American Federation of State, County, and Municipal Employees (AFSCME).

Potent factors in the anticipated success of national organizing drives in voluntary hospitals are the depressed wage structures and job conditions of these workers. According to the U.S. Department of Labor, average hourly earnings of hospital employees in March 1974 were $3.33, 73 cents an hour less than the average for manufacturing workers.

It is by examining the pay of hospital service workers that one gets a fuller picture of wages in this field. According to the 1970 United States census, the average male food service hospital worker earned just over $4000 a year while his female counterpart averaged just over $3000 a year. Male cleaning workers earned $4300 and females $3200. Clerical workers were also low earners with females averaging $4000 a year. It should be noted that in urban areas most hospital service workers are members of minority groups and 80 per cent of them are women. Whether they are men or women, black or white, the plain fact is that most hospital workers have one thing in common—they are poor.

17

On the other hand, the health care industry today is big business, employing more than four times the number of workers in the basic steel industry. More than $100 billion will be spent on health care in 1974, up from $12 billion in 1950. The nation's 7500 health care institutions employ 2.1 million workers, two-thirds of whom work in voluntary institutions. According to William Mirengoff, chairman of the government's interdepartmental committee on health manpower, the health service field will soon be the second largest, if not the largest employer in the country. The industry's growth will be further stimulated by passage of national health insurance legislation now pending in Congress.

POOR REPRESENTATION OF WORKERS IN DECISION MAKING

Another factor contributing to the big business nature of the industry lies in the composition of the boards of trustees of voluntary hospitals. Some of the most prestigious figures of American industry and finance sit on these bodies directing management of the institutions and calling the shots on labor policy. It is the social, economic, and political power wielded by these groups within hospital management that has for so long retarded organization of hospital workers.

A good illustration of the power colossus that sits on the hospital boards of trustees is the city of Pittsburgh, the heart of the steel industry. Reporting from that city during 1199's organizing campaign in 1970, Murray Kempton (1) wrote:

> Six members of the Presbyterian Hospital's board are also directors of the Mellon National Bank; two are leading officers of the Aluminum Company of America; the Presbyterian's representative is an attachment of the Mellon family. Mercy Hospital has on its board four pillars of Mellon properties, an exact balance with four nuns who represent the order the Church has charged with its administration. Negroes have been noticed with one person on the board of each hospital. Yet unions, whose health and welfare funds provide both institutions with their largest single revenue source, cannot show a solitary trustee. The management of Pittsburgh's social property rests as entirely as it ever did in the hands that own its social property.

BACKGROUND OF LOW LEVEL OF UNIONIZATION
AND THE FIRST BREAKTHROUGH

The labor movement in the United States, organized along craft lines until the great organizing drives of the CIO in the 1930s, shunned the organization of the huge work force staffing the country's voluntary hospitals. Its failure, and in some cases its refusal, to venture into the field can be attributed to a number of factors:

- Hospital employees, among the lowest paid workers in the country, were poor. Their organization would hardly swell union treasuries.
- Hospitals are widely dispersed in thousands of communities and the work force is further divided into numerous departments within each hospital, making organization more difficult.
- Federal laws excluded hospital workers from collective bargaining.
- Without the basic right to organize and with the strike weapon both illegal and frowned upon by a public concerned with helpless patients, a hospital union would have little or no clout.

- A large number of the workers were blacks, Spanish-speaking people, and members of other minority groups. To organize these workers and fight to improve their living standards required a crusading spirit.
- The power structure represented by hospital trustees presented an awesome obstacle to organization.

The first major breakthrough in hospital organization took place in New York in 1958 when District 1199 (then the 6000-member Retail Drug Employees, Local 1199) undertook the task. Two full-time organizers, Elliott Godoff and Ted Mitchell, were assigned to the campaign. New York's hospital workers then earned as little as $28 and 30 for a 44- and 48-hour, six-day week. There was no job security, little chance for advancement, no protective legislation. These workers were denied collective bargaining rights, disability benefits, unemployment insurance, and minimum wage protection. Many thousands of full-time workers had to seek supplementary assistance from welfare agencies to care for their families.

Leaning heavily on the voluntary organizing efforts of pharmacists and other drug store workers and the funds they provided, 1199 broke through by winning a consent election at Montefiore Hospital. The victory electrified the city's long-despairing hospital workers. In a three-month period, 6000 workers joined the union. Refusal by hospital managements of the union's request for representation elections released the pent-up anger of the cooks, dishwashers, nurses' aides, janitors, clerks, plumbers, and laundry workers who provided the needed services in the institutions. On May 8, 1959, 3500 "forgotten workers" at seven New York hospitals commenced a bitter 46-day strike.

The strike resulted in only a partial victory for the workers. Wage increases of $5 a week, a 40-hour week, and time-and-a-half pay for overtime were won, but still there was no union contract. But it was a beginning. The strike brought to the public an awareness of the plight of the hospital workers. And it reaffirmed the determination of the union and the workers to continue the fight for recognition. In 1962, a 56-day strike at two large hospitals saw the union's president jailed for 30 days for "contempt of court" for refusing to call off the struggle. An integral part of the settlement of this walkout was the passage of state legislation which finally gave New York City hospital workers collective bargaining rights. This law set up machinery for compulsory arbitration of disputes and outlawed hospital strikes. The law, originally limited to city hospitals, was extended statewide following another 56-day strike at Lawrence Hospital in Bronxville. The union, which had conducted the strikes to win the right to organize and bargain with the employers, had achieved its main goal.

RELATIONSHIP TO THE CIVIL RIGHTS MOVEMENT

The struggles also developed a lasting relationship with the civil rights movement, an alliance of "union power and soul power" which combined 1199's struggle to better hospital workers' economic conditions with the battle against the cause of these conditions—exploitation of the poor and discrimination against the minority groups in our society. This was expressed in an eloquent statement written in 1959, two years before the civil rights sit-in struggles took place in the South, by the late Dr. Martin Luther King Jr., an early supporter of our union:

The hospital workers' struggle is more than a fight for union rights. It is part and parcel of the larger fight in our community against discrimination and exploitation, against slums, against juvenile delinquency, against drug addiction—against all forms of degradation that result from poverty and human misery. It is a fight for human rights and human dignity.

Dr. King's statement was issued by the Committee for Justice to Hospital Workers, a coalition of 235 Black and Puerto Rican community leaders including A. Philip Randolph, Roy Wilkins, James Farmer, Whitney Young Jr., Dorothy Height, Bayard Rustin, Malcolm X, and Joseph Monserrat.

The perception of the link between the economic struggle and the struggle for human rights, and the ability to put together a coalition of the underprivileged, has been a key factor in 1199's successful organization of hospital workers.

The passage of the New York State law resulted in intensified organization of hospital service employees in the union's Hospital Division, headed by Doris Turner, a former dietary worker at Lenox Hill Hospital. Ms. Turner also serves as secretary of 1199's National Union.

TECHNICAL AND PROFESSIONAL WORKERS BEGIN TO BE ORGANIZED

A major weakness in 1199's campaign to organize hospital workers came to the forefront during the 1959 and 1962 strikes, namely the absence of technical and professional workers from the union's ranks. During the strikes the hospitals were able to continue functioning—though with great difficulty—by using supervisors and volunteers to do the cleaning, cooking, and laundry and to run the elevators. But so long as the technical staffs (x-ray, laboratory, licensed practical nurses, and other professionals) remained on the job, the hospitals could continue to operate.

It was therefore in the interest of the service workers that the technical and professional staffs be organized into 1199. This campaign was undertaken in 1964 with the formation of 1199's Guild of Professional, Technical, and Clerical Employees directed by Jesse Olson, a former pharmacist. The organization of these kinds of workers provided these employees with the benefits of union membership and immeasurably strengthened the bargaining position of all other workers in the hospitals.

Incidentally, 1199 was able to draw heavily on its early experiences as a drug store workers' union in its Guild organizing effort. The drug union had a long record of success in organizing professionals and uniting professionals and service workers into a single united organization.

Today, District 1199 represents 62,000 members in New York City and its environs, New Jersey and Connecticut.

A NATIONAL EFFORT BEGINS

The rapid progress of New York's hospital workers under 1199 leadership was watched closely by hospital workers in other cities and towns along the Eastern Seaboard and in the Midwest, and was to lead to the founding of the National Union of Hospital and Health Care Employees at the end of 1969.

New York hospital workers in 1199's Hospital and Guild Divisions, whose organization had been made possible by a small force of committed drug store workers ten years earlier, now joined with the Drug Division to provide funds and organizers for the National Union drive. The campaign was directed by National Union Executive Vice

President Elliott Godoff, aided by Henry Nicholas, a former hospital worker who is now the National Union's secretary-treasurer.

From the outset it was apparent that the road to national organization would not be smooth. The right to organize and bargain with hospital managements had to be won in some cases through the passage of laws in state legislatures or through municipal ordinances in others, or by resorting to the ultimate weapon, the strike.

The big test for the drive was not long in coming. In the spring of 1969, 500 workers, mostly black women earning $1.30 an hour, walked off their jobs in two Charleston, South Carolina hospitals, one run by the state, the other by the county. The bitter, 113-day strike in which 1000 persons, including 1199's president and the Reverend Ralph Abernathy, were jailed, shook the stately city of the Old South to its foundations and further solidified the alliance between the union and the civil rights movement. Union power and soul power, forged under the fixed bayonets of National Guardsmen patrolling the streets of Charleston, produced what the *Richmond Times-Dispatch* termed "an unbeatable combination." As Andrew J. Young, then Executive Vice President of the Southern Christian Leadership Conference (SCLC) and now a member of Congress from Georgia, told the *Dispatch*: "We worked hand in glove with the union. They didn't know their way around the South. We didn't know our way around a labor dispute. We needed each other."

Despite the fact that South Carolina, by law, doesn't bargain with labor unions, the settlement provided the workers with pay raises ranging from 30 to 70 cents an hour, with a credit union which gave them a method to deduct union dues from their paychecks, and with a grievance procedure; all in all, this meant de facto union recognition.

Mrs. Claire G. Browne, one of the strikers, commenting on the long struggle, put it this way: "It helped me to realize how important I am as a person, which I'm afraid I didn't quite realize before. I further realized that the power structure isn't all-powerful but that they are there to do the bidding of the people, and the people can make them do it."

Another result of the strike was the election, for the first time since Reconstruction, of black office holders in South Carolina.

It was on the picket lines of the Charleston strike that Coretta Scott King, Dr. King's widow and honorary chairman of 1199's national organizing drive, Walter Reuther, the late president of the United Auto Workers Union, and many other prominent labor and civil rights leaders helped to make the blue and white 1199 cap a symbol of freedom for the whole country.

The Charleston victory set the stage for the organization of 7500 service employees in Baltimore. Confronted by union organizers and with the Charleston experience fresh in mind, the Johns Hopkins Medical Center agreed to a representation election which the union won by 2 to 1. Wages rose from $1.60 an hour to $2.10. Progress was also made in Philadelphia and a number of other Pennsylvania cities. Following passage of an Act by the Pennsylvania legislature, bringing collective bargaining rights to hospital workers (a result of 1199's threat to strike Presbyterian Hospital), the union won more than 20 representation elections covering 7000 workers.

Elaborate anti-union campaigns by some hospital managements have created an image of 1199 ferocity that does not conform to the facts. A look at the record shows that the union has seldom, if ever, conducted a strike which resulted from a breakdown or disagreement in negotiations. Rarely has 1199 conducted strikes or stoppages over wage or other economic items generally included in collective bargaining agreements.

Practically all of 1199's strikes have been over the right to union recognition and would not have taken place if there had been adequate collective bargaining legislation covering hospital workers.

BENEFITS OF UNIONIZATION

Established along the East Coast and building a base in Wisconsin, Michigan, Ohio, Virginia, and West Virginia, the National Union is transforming the lives of hospital workers. It has demonstrated to those living in poverty that they can rise from it and make better lives for themselves and their children. In 16 years New York hospital workers in 1199 have seen wages rise from $28-30 a week to the current minimum of $171 in the lowest paid jobs. This minimum will rise to $181 on July 1, 1975.

The 1199 National Union Benefit Fund provides members and their families with extensive hospital, medical, and laboratory care at no cost to the member. Dental and prescription drug coverage is also provided. Each year, the union sends members' children to summer camp for three weeks, at no cost to the parents. In the summer of 1974, 308 youngsters from five states attended six camps in New York, New Jersey, and Vermont. Also each year 200 members' children chosen primarily on the basis of need are the recipients of college scholarship funds.

To be effective, the organization of hospital workers must be accompanied by the development of programs designed to weld together working people differing in color, religion, educational background, and political beliefs into a fighting organization capable of defending itself on a day-to-day basis on the job.

An educational program sponsored by 1199 does more than train union leadership at all levels. A training and upgrading program which takes thousands of workers from dead-end jobs and trains them for more highly skilled hospital employment has been established. The program, financed by employer contributions of one per cent of payroll, leads to upgrading to practical nurse; lab, x-ray, and surgical technician; respiratory inhalation therapist; registered nurse; and other, more responsible, hospital jobs.

A $30 million New York City urban renewal project sponsored by 1199 has been completed on the Harlem bank of the East River. The 1590-unit cooperative housing project includes many union members and their families. The project, on a 9.5-acre riverfront tract, has the most modern facilities for community living and recreation, including a medical center, child day-care center, swimming pool, gymnasium, sauna bath, and landscaped grounds and play areas. In an appraisal of the project in the *New York Times* on November 2, 1974, Paul Goldberger, the paper's architectural writer, termed it "superb" and "one of New York's most architecturally significant housing projects."

THE BROADER SOCIAL GOAL OF THE UNION

It is the goal of 1199 to build a democratic organization that relies on its rank-and-file and calls for maximum involvement of hospital workers in the effort not only to improve working conditions, but to change social conditions so that all will have a better life. This calls for increased participation of hospital employees in the city, state, and federal political process. For years 1199 was among the few trade unions actively opposed to the war in Vietnam, and the union played a decisive role in mobilizing opposition to the war within the labor movement.

District 1199 was the first union to actively oppose wage controls. In November 1973, when the Cost of Living Council set aside the wage increases that were due its members in a contract reached through binding arbitration, this action precipitated the biggest hospital strike in the nation's history, involving 35,000 workers at 62 hospitals.

Whenever 1199's National Union undertakes a hospital organizing drive in a new area, hospital management reacts in typical fashion. Labor relations specialists are called in. Public relations experts are hired. Wage increases are announced. The hospital director issues regular bulletins emphasizing the management's keen interest in the workers' problems. Invariably, the phrase, "my door is always open," appears in one or more such statements.

Along with this propaganda barrage, the management will usually conduct a private investigation of 1199 and its officers. A team of management experts will visit New York, talk to management representatives who have contacts with 1199, and will draft a confidential report which is circulated among directors and trustees in the area under organization. For the most part it is typical anti-union stuff, but it often contains considerable truth.

Here, for example, are excerpts from a document on 1199 which was circulated among hospital directors in a large urban area.

- The leadership of Local 1199 is idealistic and honest ... [they] take relatively low pay, pay their staff at such low levels that money doesn't hold them, only dedication. There are no shakedowns, gifts, entertainment or under the table deals of any kind between management and the staff of the union.
- The union syphons off loyalty from the hospital. One technique is to involve the workers in social and political causes.
- The union trains its stewards well on such matters as the grievance procedure.
- The union's techniques in organizing New York City's hospitals were successful because of the leadership's ability in involving support from civil rights and other groups outside the hospitals.
- Both in their organizing campaign in New York and their life under labor contracts, this union has demonstrated that it is one of the most militant—most demanding—most difficult unions in America to deal with. However, unlike some of the other militant longshore and teamster unions, this union is not corrupt.
- Many of the confrontations and work stoppages relate to actions of unwise supervisors. Dignity of the worker is a term most frequently used in disputes. All supervisors have had either to respond to training in supervisory practices or to be fired.
- The hospitals in New York are surviving with Local 1199 and the hospitals in this city can survive.... This union will force good supervisory practices upon the institutions.

CONCLUSION

It is clear to us that the organization of hospital workers into a national union is going to take place. Obviously, it will take lots of hard work. In the final analysis it will depend on the readiness and willingness of these workers to fight to put an end to poverty wages and win a measure of respect and dignity on the job.

There is a huge mural on the front of District 1199's headquarters in New York City. It depicts health care employees on the job, at home, and at play. In the center is a statement from the black abolitionist leader, Frederick Douglass. That statement tells what our union is all about. It says: "If there is no struggle there can be no progress."

REFERENCE

1. Kempton, M. *New York Review of Books*, April 9, 1970.

CHAPTER 4

Unionization, Strikes, Threatened Strikes, And Hospitals: The View From Hospital Management

Robert K. Match, Arnold H. Goldstein, and Harold L. Light

THE DEVELOPMENT OF UNIONS IN HOSPITALS

Although the first hospital employee union was recognized more than 50 years ago, there were only scattered instances of collective bargaining in hospitals prior to the 1960s. Recently, however, hospital administrators and trustees have expressed concern over the rapid increase of unionization of hospital employees. Their concern has been motivated by the extent of collective bargaining activities, the rate of union expansion, the number and effects of work stoppages, and the impact of unionization upon the hospital's ability to function and on the management of its finances and resources.

Historically, union organizing efforts and the recognition of unions have moved at a rather slow pace. The recent rapid growth of unions in all segments of the hospital work force is attributed to many factors. These include a national drive to organize hospital workers mounted by various unions throughout the United States in 1959, the inadequacy of hospital management policies regarding personnel, including policies on wages and increments, the lack of grievance machinery and of proper supervision, the general absence of effective employee communication and participation, and the economic and political forces that have shaped the financing of health services in the 1970s.

Labor's position was expressed by Nelson H. Cruikshank, Director of the Department of Social Security of the AFL-CIO, in the July 1959 issue of *The Modern Hospital* (1):

> Organized labor often speaks of "democracy in the workplace." To its millions of members, this phrase can be translated to mean a voice in working conditions and a sense of human dignity and respect on the job .... It is hard to believe that any carefully considered "principle" can serve to deny these hospital employees the same rights presently enjoyed by millions of other American workers.

Unionism has, in effect, provided the employee with a voice in the determination of wages, hours, and personnel practices. It has also provided the employee with a sense of security and strength in numbers, and has helped employees feel that there is a skilled organization to represent them.

In an article entitled "Nation's Hospitals Face Union Drive," in the same issue of *The Modern Hospital,* an additional factor in labor's organizing efforts in the hospitals was noted (2):

> Many observers believed the nation's top union leaders had become alarmed because membership in the huge industrial unions had been declining in recent years, with a resulting loss in union revenues. "The hospital working force is a rich, new source of dues-paying union members, if it can be developed," an industrialist told a group of hospital administrators at one of the 1959 hospital conventions.

Unions are always seeking new members; the labor force has doubled from 40 million, 35 years ago, to some 88 million today, and the size of the increased labor pool is viewed by unions as a fresh resource for their organizing efforts. They feel that they should organize the unorganized in all areas, but especially view the health care industry as fertile territory for their efforts because it may conceivably become the largest single employer among the industries of the United States. Competition among unions for members from the hospitals also exists. Thus, the Garment Workers, Meat Packers, Teamsters, the Service Workers International Union, the American Federation of State, County and Municipal Workers, the Communications Workers of America, the National Union of Hospital and Health Care Employees, and others all have organized hospital workers (3).

Minority groups have also become more militant and involved and have recognized collective bargaining as a method for equalizing relationships.

The pathway to unionization in the hospital field started basically with federal employees, progressed to state, municipal, and proprietary employees, and finally reached those in the nonprofit sector, the only sector previously exempt from labor laws, except in states which had passed such legislation. Because recent amendments to the Taft-Hartley Law have now removed this exemption, a huge potential membership pool has been opened, in the labor-intensive, not-for-profit health care facilities. These facilities employ an estimated 1.5 million workers, only 12 per cent of whom are now unionized.

Once the national campaign to organize hospital workers was mounted, the unions concentrated their efforts mainly on nonprofessional workers, whose wages and working conditions were totally inadequate. For example, in 1959, the lowest hiring scale for unskilled workers in a hospital in New York City was $147 a month or approximately $35 per week (4). It is important to point out, however, that even while employees were receiving such low wages, some voluntary hospitals in New York City were incurring operating deficits. These deficits came about because sources of support for patient services did not provide adequate reimbursement to the institutions and because the great advances made in medical technology required more expensive equipment and skilled personnel. There is no doubt that hospital workers were in essence bearing the burden of the inadequate financing and were in fact subsidizing hospital operations.

While present patterns of formal bargaining are partly a function of hospital size, the distribution of union recognition by region illustrates that other forces also are involved. One important factor has been the laws regulating labor relations. The

National Labor Relations Act (Wagner Act) was one such law. Passed in 1935, it did not specifically exclude nonprofit hospitals, and, in 1944, a Federal Court affirmed the National Labor Relations Board's jurisdiction over hospitals (5). However, in 1947, the Taft-Hartley amendments to the federal law excluded from its coverage corporations or associations operating a hospital, if no part of the net earnings inured to the benefit of any private shareholder or individual (6). In 1967, the National Labor Relations Board asserted jurisdiction over proprietary hospitals and nursing homes even though the Board had, historically, refused such jurisdiction.

In reversing its former position, the Board found that proprietary hospitals with gross revenues of $250,000 would, in fact, affect interstate commerce because skilled personnel were obtained from outside the local area, and such hospitals were no longer charitable because of the presence of the third-party payors. A mechanism was also provided to prevent recognition strikes, with the Board stating that hospital employees should have the same rights to collective bargaining as others. In addition, the Board ruled that nursing homes operated in a similar fashion to proprietary hospitals and so accepted jurisdiction over facilities that received annual gross revenues of $100,000 or more (7).

Several states also enacted their own labor relations laws. In each of ten states, nongovernmental nonprofit hospitals are now included under the provisions of the statute, which generally requires collective bargaining recognition.

What happened in federal hospitals is an example of this regulatory influence. The unusual level of collective bargaining in federal hospitals since 1967 can be attributed almost entirely to an executive order issued five years earlier. Prior to 1962, federal employees did not have the right to bargain collectively, but an executive order issued in that year by President John F. Kennedy established collective bargaining rights for federal employees, including those in federal hospitals.

An important factor in the increase of collective bargaining in hospitals has been the extent of collective bargaining generally in an area. If a large part of the area's work force is unionized, hospital employees in that area are prone to organize in order to obtain additional income or benefits. It is probable that the public response to unions is more favorable in such areas than in areas of low union membership.

Table 1

Extent of collective bargaining contracts in hospitals
in 1961, 1967, and 1970 by control of hospital[a]

Control	1961		1967		1970	
	Total Number of Registered Hospitals	Percentage with Contracts	Total Number of Registered Hospitals	Percentage with Contracts	Total Number of Registered Hospitals	Percentage with Contracts
All hospitals	6,923	3.0	7,172	7.7	7,123	14.7
Federal	437	0.0	416	22.6	408	52.0
Nonfederal	6,486	3.2	2,141 [sic]	6.8	6,715	12.4
Nongovernmental not-for-profit	3,588	4.3	3,692	8.2	3,600	12.4
For-profit	973	4.3	923	4.9	858	8.0
State and local	1,925	1.0	2,141	5.3	2,257	14.1

[a]Source, reference 8.

Table 2

Extent of collective bargaining contracts and requests for collective bargaining recognition in
hospitals in 1967 and 1970 by bed size and census division[a]

	1967			1970		
Categorization	Total Number of Registered Hospitals	Percentage with Contracts	Percentage with Requests	Total Number of Registered Hospitals	Percentage with Contracts	Percentage with Requests
All hospitals	7,172	7.7	5.2	7,123	14.7	3.7
Bed size category						
6- 24	542	1.3	0.7	447	2.2	0.7
25- 49	1,629	2.4	1.0	1,475	4.3	0.7
50- 99	1,734	5.4	2.6	1,713	8.5	1.8
100-199	1,365	8.9	5.3	1,473	14.7	3.7
200-299	686	14.0	9.3	698	25.2	5.9
300-399	375	14.7	12.5	427	24.2	7.3
400-499	220	15.5	14.1	261	33.7	9.6
500+	621	17.4	14.7	629	38.6	11.0
Division						
New England	415	5.8	8.7	414	21.7	5.1
Middle Atlantic	896	11.4	7.4	888	25.0	6.3
South Atlantic	925	3.4	4.1	949	7.8	3.1
East North Central	1,169	8.7	8.6	1,132	17.6	6.7
East South Central	551	3.4	2.5	534	5.6	2.1
West North Central	901	9.2	2.7	903	11.3	1.9
West South Central	956	1.4	1.6	940	3.8	0.5
Mountain	441	4.3	4.1	438	8.9	3.9
Pacific	918	17.6	6.3	925	27.5	3.6

[a]Source, reference 8.

The American Hospital Association surveyed the extent of collective bargaining in hospitals in 1961, 1967, and 1970 (8). Findings from the 1970 study clearly indicate that the extent and rate of unionization continues to increase (see Table 1). As with other sectors of the economy, union organizing in the hospital sector tends to occur in larger work units. Table 2 indicates that the bed size of hospitals is a factor in explaining both the extent and growth of collective bargaining in hospitals (9).

ORGANIZATION OF PROFESSIONALS

Employee organization in collective bargaining, while clearly established in the American labor movement, did not directly affect the health professionals until recently when some groups began to concern themselves with the need to organize; dissatisfaction regarding their own position in relation to insurers, hospitals, and government, and trends in the economy, have been greatly responsible for health professionals beginning to organize.

In 1967, the AFL-CIO Council for Professional, Scientific, and Cultural Employees was established by nine international unions to facilitate the organization of 10 million nonunion professional employees in the United States and special emphasis was placed on organizing employees in the hospital sector (10).

Professional associations are also actively involved in trying to upgrade and negotiate terms and conditions for their memberships. The American Nurses Association (ANA), for instance, has long sought economic protection and other advantages for the nursing professional. In 1937 the ANA recommended that nurses not join unions and suggested that they work to improve their professional situation through the Association. In 1946, the house of delegates of the ANA officially initiated an economic security program and urged that all state and district nurses' associations push this program vigorously and expeditiously (11).

By January 1974 475 contracts had been negotiated by 33 state nurses' associations, covering approximately 65,000 registered nurses and including 381 contracts negotiated in 11 states with labor laws that protect the rights of nurses to enter into collective bargaining units.

As with nonprofessionals, organized labor has also encouraged the organization of professional employees because of the potential membership pool that they offer. Professional employees are now faced with the choice of affiliating with their professional associations or with trade unions. The complicating factor for the professional is the fear that his appropriate interests may not be completely protected in units in which he is greatly outnumbered by nonprofessional employees; in some instances, there is the added philosophical conflict about the ethical propriety of union membership.

The Committee of Interns and Residents, which at present is not formally affiliated within the trade union movement, has had correspondence with George Meany, President of the AFL-CIO, on the subject of unionization. Practicing physicians are interested in influencing the climate in which medicine is practiced as well as the income they receive from it. Complaints have been registered that income has not kept pace with the cost of practicing medicine and that third-party payors are telling physicians how to practice. According to a recent article (12), William L. Kircher, Director of Organization for the AFL-CIO, "has a sympathetic attitude toward the principle of doctors' unionization." However, he does not feel that doctors will be able to use collective bargaining to get a fair economic break from the government and other third parties unless they become employees of those parties.

Mr. Kircher is aware that doctors, in the past, have denounced unions, even though now they are talking about, and actually forming their own union. He understands that they realize there is strength in unionism and their previous feelings about unions could very well be dissipated by what they see as their present unfavorable environment (12).

A recent national survey taken among physicians indicated that three of every five doctors believe they should unionize (12). The survey also found that a number of doctors would be willing to turn to professional labor leaders. Another survey indicated that if they considered it necessary, more than half the doctors responding would strike—provided that emergency services were not interrupted (12).

MANAGEMENT'S VIEW TOWARD
UNIONIZATION OF HOSPITAL WORKERS

Hospital trustees and administrators have been deeply concerned about the possible effects of unionization upon already difficult hospital operations and, with several exceptions, they have opposed the organization of hospital workers. Many questions were posed which dealt with management's concern as to whether union activities might so interfere with management that hospital operations would be made more difficult than they already are. They have argued that charitable nonprofit hospitals are not a legitimate area for union organizational efforts because the objectives of these institutions are social rather than economic (13). Deep concern has been expressed about the possible impact of strikes and slowdowns upon patient care, and such actions have been labeled as irresponsible, since the basic stakes are not income distribution but human life (13). With increased labor costs, the already underfinanced not-for-profit hospitals were further inhibited in expansion of programs and services because of the increased competition for a limited number of dollars. Regardless of the concerns expressed by management, however, strikes have occurred, employees in hospitals have been organized, and a new era of collective bargaining in the hospital industry has begun.

COLLECTIVE BARGAINING

According to Davey (14),

> Collective bargaining is defined as a continuing institutional relationship between an employer entity and a labor organization representing exclusively a defined group of employees concerned with the negotiation, administration, interpretation and enforcement of written agreements covering joint understanding as to wages or salaries, rates of pay, hours of work, and other conditions of employment.

In 1959, Ray Amberg, President of the American Hospital Association, wrote of collective bargaining as follows (15):

> Collective bargaining has arisen as a desire for a democratic method to solve the problems of employer-employee relations principally due to the lack of proper functioning of the direct employer-employee method .... But we no longer possess the right in many cases to deny our workers the privilege of collective bargaining provided they feel that the old system is unjust, unfair, or for any other reason not in their best interest.

The problem with collective bargaining in hospitals is that where strong hospital unions exist it is difficult to accommodate the interests of employees, payors, patients, and hospitals because of the pressure that such unions can exert to support their demands. The difference between nonprofit hospitals and private enterprises is that competitive, product-market forces do not confront the former. Product-market forces, in effect, can restrain large settlements at the bargaining table because of the impact they could have on sales and competition, which could possibly result in unemployment. Such market restrictions do not apply to the not-for-profit hospitals, where the vast portion of hospital operating revenue depends on third-party payors which, in essence, means that organized consumers and intermediaries can participate in decisions that pertain to the organization, delivery, and cost of health services.

Ronald L. Miller (16) has said that the "cost-pass-through" mechanism of insurance financing and government assistance programs, which makes sure that negotiated labor increases are passed through to third-party reimbursers, "gives the payors direct interest in the decisions made at the bargaining table." However, as Miller points out,

> Confronting the hospital are present and potential constraints on the use of the cost-pass-through mechanism. These constraints are political forces, rather than product-market forces; they are reflected in the increasing role of governmental and quasi-governmental agencies in the hospital managerial function. Furthermore, without product-market forces to limit hospital cost increases, payors will have to protect their economic interest through direct participation in the hospital managerial function and by lobbying for government regulatory control. In either case, the absence of market forces makes hospital collective bargaining a multiparty process, in contrast to the traditional bipartite character of private enterprise collective bargaining. In industries that are dependent upon government subsidies for continued operation or in which product-market forces are evaluated as not protecting the so-called "public interest," the multiparty character of collective bargaining is increasingly evident. . . .
>
> The growing number of internal and external participants in the hospital managerial function raises a critical question: with whom should hospital unions negotiate? In an institution with strong employee organizations and regulated hospital income, hospital management is a middleman in the bargaining that takes place between those who finance hospital care and the employees who provide the services. For example, negotiations between the League of Voluntary Hospitals, New York City, and Local 1199 are fundamentally between state officials and a powerful union. An accord must be struck between increasing payroll costs and increasing insurance premiums and subsidies. . . .
>
> A recurrent theme in the literature on hospital collective bargaining is that strikes result primarily from the lack of alternate methods to resolve the issue of representation. This premise concludes that, should hospital employees be accorded representation election rights, the occurrence of work stoppages would be minimized. The record of the past decade does not fully support such a conclusion. Strike activity during the 1950s and in the mid-1960s was primarily organizational. During the past five years, however, an increasing number of legal and illegal work stoppages have resulted from bargaining impasses.

STRIKES

Strikes have often been used as a weapon to resolve labor disputes. In private industry, most conflicts which arise in the formulation of a new contract may be resolved by a test of bargaining power, including the use of the strike. This test is deemed an essential ingredient of the collective bargaining process. But disputes in industry rarely have an impact on life and death. In the health care sector, where patient care and welfare is jeopardized, there has been ample demonstration that even where it has been specifically illegal for hospital employees to strike, the strike weapon has been used. An example of this is the series of strikes by District 1199 against hospitals in New York. Labor leaders have contended that as labor-management relationships in the hospital industry mature, there will be fewer strikes.

Strikes against the voluntary hospitals in New York City have been, perhaps by far, the most critical and publicized labor disputes in the entire hospital industry; these have occurred in violation of pledges not to strike made by the union, and have continued even after the courts have ordered the strikers to return to work.

An official of District 1199 of the National Union of Hospital and Health Care Employees had indicated that "it was never their aim to make a strike 100 per cent effective. They wanted a strike to be effective enough to make a hospital capitulate rather than evacuate (17)." Another official of District 1199 was also quoted as saying that strikes were a thing of the past in New York State: "Now that all of the state is covered by progressive hospital labor law," he said, "the days of hospital strikes in the state are over—unqualifiedly (17)."

Yet, in spite of these previous no-strike assurances, in 1973 the 48 member hospitals of the League of Voluntary Homes and Hospitals in New York City (which accounted for about half of the hospital beds in the city) were crippled by an eight-day strike by 30,000 District 1199 employees that severely curtailed the services at these hospitals and nursing homes.

This strike resulted from the Cost of Living Council's failure to come to a decision on a 7.5 per cent pay and benefit increase. The strike continued in the face of a $500,000 fine to the union, and a personal fine to its officers, and even after the City's Health Department had declared a state of emergency.

The League of Voluntary Homes and Hospitals estimated that 12,000 of the 23,000 beds at the 48 institutions were emptied as patients were discharged or transferred to other institutions. During the strike, hospitals shut down all outpatient clinics and permitted only emergency admissions. At least two hospitals closed services entirely. Pickets prevented garbage pick-up, and at 43 institutions the accumulated waste was declared a fire and health hazard. Acts of violence at the picket line occurred, with as many as 22 persons arrested in a single day.

As Miller (18) has pointed out, the right to strike generally given to employees in private industry has not been readily given to hospital employees because it has been amply demonstrated that work stoppages have an impact on the availability of patient services. The threat of strike and the strike itself in the health care sector provide a disproportionate amount of coercive power that can be placed in the hands of a strong union.

Miller believes that, as a method of resolving disputes, the strike is basically inconsistent with both the economic characteristics and the service objectives of hospitals. The consequences of nonagreement between a strongly organized union and a hospital fall primarily upon the public. Miller (18) continues by stating that:

> The ability of the hospital and striking employees to endure economic losses is not relevant in the manner that is normally associated with the costs of work stoppages in private enterprise . . . . In private enterprise, a strike performs its function of inducing concessions from both union and management if the employees and the firm suffer economic losses and if the primary impact of the strike is upon the employees and the firm. For an increasing number of private sector industries, as for not-for-profit hospitals political tolerance of the strike becomes a relevant question when the primary and immediate impact of the strike is upon third-party or public interests. Political considerations relate both to disruptions in the availability of essential services and to the impact of negotiations upon patient charges. Tactics for manipulating political intervention are integral elements in the use or threat of legal and illegal work stoppages. Indeed, it has not been uncommon for hospitals to take a firm position in negotiations, with the intent of placing responsibility upon the government and the union for subsequent cost increases . . . . Whether union participation without the strike is meaningful largely depends upon the degree to which substitute procedures are acceptable to the various parties of direct interest.

ALTERNATIVES

There are several alternatives to the strike in the process of collective bargaining. These include fact-finding, voluntary arbitration, and compulsory arbitration. With the exception of compulsory arbitration, these alternatives are largely dependent upon the agreement of both parties. Fact finding is not binding upon the parties and both have the right to accept or reject the recommendations. In the use of voluntary arbitration, both the union and management can start the process, determine the issues, and select the panel. Compulsory arbitration, in the view of some experts, is detrimental to the bargaining process because both parties have no choice in the matter. The effect of compulsory arbitration in the Minneapolis-St. Paul area was noted as follows:

> In contrast to New York City, the availability of compulsory arbitration procedures has shaped contractual provisions in Minneapolis-St. Paul. During the past 22 years contracts between Local 113 (Hospital and Institutional Employees Union) and the Twin City Hospital Association have been determined in large measure through compulsory arbitration. The dependence of Local 113 and the hospital association upon arbitration of new contract terms is one result of a poor working relationship between the two parties. Their contracts have been a cumbersome accumulation of arbitrated provisions. The parties have had little success in clarifying the agreements through direct negotiations and have come to accept new contract arbitration as standard practice. These deficiencies notwithstanding, the hospitals have been essentially free of work stoppages.

Experience in the San Francisco Bay area would suggest that extensive influence by third-party interests upon union-hospital negotiations can be an important element for stable collective bargaining under voluntary arbitration. During the 1940s, the San Francisco City Labor Council was largely responsible for bringing about recognition of Local 250 (Hospital and Institutional Workers Union) by San Francisco hospitals, and the Council has since influenced the conduct of hospital collective bargaining. However, militants within the Local have charged that the Council's concern with charges and services restrains economic gains that could be accomplished with greater coercive pressures applied by the union. The aggressiveness of the California State Nurses Association, which was involved in a lengthy strike in the San Francisco Bay area in 1974, may have undermined the apparent stability of collective bargaining enjoyed by all parties concerned.

CONCLUSION

Hospital unions have derived great benefits from the arbitration process because of both the way in which arbitration panels have been selected and the influence of local and state politicians upon settlements which have traditionally been supported through the mechanism of cost-pass-throughs. Confronted by new union contracts, inflationary contract settlements, and regulatory confinements, and confounded in their attempts to regulate cost increases because of fear of government control reprisals, increasingly hospitals have had to scrape for their economic viability. Many such institutions are bankrupt or on the verge of bankruptcy. While hospital management would like to see employee wages determined with reference to both economics and patient care, the collective bargaining process at the local level has not always been satisfactory to the hospital's position. Arbitration awards should be made by arbitrators who have no local vested interest in the settlement. Accordingly, arbitrators should be appointed from outside of the local region. Because of the catastrophic nature of strikes upon the care and welfare of patients, as well as upon employees, the arbitration award should be binding upon both parties and should be federally enforced.

REFERENCES

1. Cruikshank, N. H. The case for the unionization of hospital workers. *Mod. Hosp.* 93(1): 71-72, 1959.
2. Nation's hospitals face union drive. *Mod. Hosp.* 93(1): 61-62, 1959.
3. *A Directory of Public Employees Organizations. A Guide to the Major Organizations Representing State and Local Public Employees,* p. 44. U.S. Department of Labor, Labor Management Service Administration, November 1971.
4. Cherkasky, M. Why we signed a union agreement. *Mod. Hosp.* 93: 64-70, July 1959.
5. Central Dispensary and Emergency Hospital. U NLRB, S7 NLRB 393, aff'd F. 2d 853 (D.C. Circ. 1944).
6. Labor Management Relations Act, 1947, 61 stat., 136, 29, U.S.C. ch. 141 sec. 2(2).
7. Graham, H. E. Effects on NLRB jurisdictional charge on union organizing activity in the proprietary health care sector, p. 278. In *Proceedings of the 24th Annual Winter Meeting, December 27-28, 1971.* Industrial Relations Research Association, 1972.
8. AHA research capsules No. 6. *Hospitals* 46: 217-218, April 1972.
9. Miller, J. D., and Shurtell, S. M. Hospital unionization: A study of the trends. *Hospitals* 43(16): 67-73, 1969.
10. Pointer, D. D., and Cannedy, L. L. Organizing of professionals. *Hospitals* 46(6): 70-73, 1972.
11. Munger, M. D. American nurses program to promote collective bargaining. *Hospital Topics* p. 21, May 1974.
12. Urlich, S. Will your appendectomy be performed by a member of the AFL-CIO? *Mod. Hosp.* 121(4): 63-67, 1973.
13. Remarks outlining the New York voluntary hospitals' position with regard to unions and threats of strikes given by Martin R. Steinberg, M. D., Director, Mount Sinai Hospital, at a meeting of voluntary hospital representatives requested by New York Commissioner of Labor Felix, April 16, 1959.
14. Davey, H. S. *Contemporary Collective Bargaining,* Ed. 3, p. 3. Prentice-Hall, New York, 1972.
15. Amberg, R. Your president reports (editorial). *Hospitals* 33(11): 51, 1959.
16. Miller, R. L. The hospital-union relationship, part 1. *Hospitals* 45(9): 49-54, 1971.
17. Carlson, D. R. Labor union: Color it white, black, or red. *Mod. Hosp.* 105(2): 107-111, 1965.
18. Miller, R. L. The hospital-union relationship, part 2. *Hospitals* 45(10): 52-56, 1971.

CHAPTER 5

The Purposes Of Unionization In The Medical Profession: The Unionized Profession's Perspective In The United States

Sanford A. Marcus

As the 20th century enters its final quarter, the tempo of socioeconomic change that has characterized this epoch has quickened immeasurably. Conflicts and accommodations between communism and capitalism, the crumbling of colonialism, various forms of authoritarianism, the assertion of the power of labor, all have been part of the cavalcade of this century. As technology and communication have advanced, the yearning for freedom and the fruits of the good life have filtered down to segments of humanity where they had never been articulated before. This has indeed become the century of the common man.

THE SEEDS OF CONFLICT

Amid these egalitarian notions there has emerged the dictum that health care is a basic human right, somewhat akin to life, liberty, and the pursuit of happiness. This has indeed been a worldwide thrust, and few countries of any degree of sophistication have failed to acknowledge its reality. In countries whose economies are basically socialistic, health care is simply one extension of the services rendered by the state to its citizens. The purveyors of this service are compensated—each according to his needs—as is proper in a socialist state, and no claim for special merit or status can be made by them. It is in those nations that still proclaim themselves to be capitalistic where the transition of health care from an entrepreneurial service to a state-controlled service is fraught with difficulty, especially where other socioeconomic class relationships are left undisturbed, and more glaringly during a period of relatively great affluence.

Historically the medical profession in the United States has been independent of regulation beyond the usual stringencies of the marketplace. The physician as healer has been accorded a place of respect and esteem by the very nature of the service he rendered—personal concern, amelioration of suffering, quasi-mystical intervention in the struggle between life and the inevitability of death, these were his stock in trade. There was the tacit acceptance of the fact that he should be accorded a special niche in society, measured both by the honor it accorded him and by a standard of living that was reasonably expected to be somewhat above others whose responsibilities were less than his. His long years of training, hours of service, risk of exposure to disease, shortened earning life-span, attenuated freedom and family life, and devotion to professional self-advancement all seemed to justify a special status. In return, the American medical profession developed a high standard of medical care that was unequaled anywhere in the world, indeed a fair exchange, it would seem.

With progressive urbanization and industrialization the role of the physician became even more important as centrifugal forces disrupted neighborhoods and families and compartmentalized life styles. He became perhaps the last bastion of personalized service, of individual concern, in an increasingly depersonalized society. Scientific advances in dramatic profusion enabled him to increase his armamentarium, to extend his range of services and achieve real breakthroughs in illnesses that had scourged mankind from the dawn of time. This was certainly the Golden Age of Medicine.

Society itself, however, began to change more rapidly. Government began to assume more and more responsibility for the vicissitudes of life, economic insecurity, illness, old age—originally in behalf of those who could not provide for their own needs, but later for all of its citizens. Conceived originally as a floor to be placed under human misery, the involvement of government has progressed to the point of assuring the good life—the guaranteed annual wage—a risk-free existence to the entire populace. Seminars on redistribution of wealth are commonplace in high government circles.

FORCES INTERPOSED BETWEEN PHYSICIAN AND PATIENT

The conflict is first perceived in the recognition that medical service, the most personal and individualized of all services, does not lend itself well to the homogenization inherent in such massive government involvement. Computerized norms, quality standards, and cost controls—so essential to a military procurement program, for example, cannot easily be applied to health care. The primary agents in health care delivery, the physicians, find themselves in the novel position of coping with all sorts of forces that are interposing themselves between them and their patients.

The Insurance Industry

The first of these is the insurance industry, which is essentially a transition phenomenon, an attempt to obtain predictability of risk, before government becomes completely involved. With the undeniable explosion in health-care costs it has become increasingly necessary for the individual to be protected from these costs, either by purchasing his own insurance, by obtaining it as a fringe benefit of his employment, or by ultimately receiving it through one or another government program. Despite the fact that only about one-seventh of these costs devolve to the personal benefit of the physicians, it is the doctors who ultimately direct and channel the allocation of most of these expenditures. Inflation, sophisticated advances in treatment, and rising expectations for more and better services on the part of the public, have increased the cost-consciousness of the insurance carriers as they will increasingly stimulate that of the government. Their conflicts with the medical profession become more acute daily.

The basic conflict between insurance carriers and the medical profession, however, is a philosophical one. Insurance is essentially a group service—the greatest good for the greatest number—while medicine, as indicated, is a one-to-one relationship. Insurance has as its ultimate goal the paying out of the minimum benefits commensurate with its premium structure, while the physician seeks the maximum benefit for his individual patient. It is here that the dispute focuses; cost considerations are pitted against medical judgment, and the positions are essentially irreconcilable. Were the insurance carriers to grant the medical profession carte blanche the companies could not operate profitably. And when physicians are compelled to involve themselves in cost control, a point of no return is reached in the degree that they can properly compromise their duty to the individual patients they serve.

The Hospital Industry

The second force that interposes itself between the physician and his patient is the hospital industry. Originally conceived as workshops where specialized functions were performed that could not be done elsewhere, the hospitals often have evolved into convenience stations where the creature-comforts of the patient could be served with reduced imposition on his family. The convenience of the physician is also served by the gathering together of several of his patients in one place with a saving of time and transportation. Again, mounting costs have sharpened the differences between the objectives of the hospital and the physicians. A frenzy of overexpansion launched in the sixties in response to a supposed shortage of hospital beds has, in fact, resulted in a glut of surplus beds. The economic embarrassment occasioned by their very existence has led to a variety of efforts to keep them occupied, and ultimately has created a struggle for power between hospital administrators and the medical profession. The hospital empires that have been built are crumbling—model "medical centers" are going bankrupt—and the legions of hospital administrators are attempting to salvage their status and their very raison d'être by grasping for control over all health care delivery during this period of great transition. They have been aided immeasurably by the habit patterns of many physicians in relying too heavily on hospitalization, and by certain legal opinions that make the lay administration of hospitals responsible for the ultimate quality of care. This illusion of dependency by physicians on hospitals has emboldened administrators to usurp the right to interpret the actual quality and modalities of health care, a circumstance that any conscientious physician must find intolerable.

The Intrusion of Government

The third and final force that is intruding into the traditional doctor-patient relationship is government. It is evident that within the next two or three years the percentage of Americans whose health care needs are financed wholly or in part by government will rise from a present 37 per cent to 100 per cent. The historical forces that have conditioned the public to accept health care as a right of citizenship assure that fact. With such massive involvement must come cost controls—the need for accountability in utilization, for example—if fiscal chaos is to be avoided. The inevitability of the conflict between these cost considerations and the human values involved in the doctor-patient relationship becomes more clear daily. The political wisdom of *not* advising the electorate that their quantity and quality of health care must be cut back by budgetary stringencies is obvious. Any citizen who perceived that he might be asked to surrender some of the individuality of his personal health care to satisfy broader social goals would be certain to rebel at the polling place next election. It is only through the devious device of an attack on the "professional standards" of the medical profession that political hay can be made, especially when the highest government officials proclaim that "physicians make too much money"—it's part of the contemporary fun and games to topple the mighty. The inevitable phasing out of private practice by direct government subsidy to other forms of practice will render all physicians totally dependent on government policy and whim within the next very few years.

MEDICAL UNIONISM IN THE
BRAVE NEW WORLD OF MEDICINE

It is at this point that we return to the position of the physician in the Brave New World of Medicine that is emerging. With the forces that are arrayed against him it becomes certain that without vigorous representation of his rights by forces that have been conspicuously lacking in the past, the physician must certainly be reduced to the level of a public functionary, accorded no more respect or status than the poor postal employees or public-school teachers in *their* pre-union days. It is fatuous and vain to hope that the value of the physician to society should be self-evident. All his posturing about professionalism becomes tragicomical when idols are toppling all around him. If he indeed feels pride in the dignity and achievements of his profession he is being called upon for the first time in history to exemplify that pride through concrete action rather than lofty rhetoric. With nostalgia for the good old days, but imbued with the pragmatic realization that *none* of his values can otherwise be preserved, he is reluctantly entering the Age of Medical Unionization.

What is a medical union and what can it hope to accomplish? Well, it is apparent that a broad spectrum of opinion and interpretation of labor history makes this a difficult question to answer without passion or prejudice. A union can be said to represent the socioeconomic interest of its members through collective action made possible by their individual commitment to its purposes. This far transcends the degree of loyalty of physicians to their professional societies, and connotes a willingness to allow the union to negotiate the best possible arrangements, and to abide by the results of that collective bargaining. At the present time the traditional union demand for "more" probably does not really apply to dollars and cents considerations for physicians. But with the almost vengeful attitude of our wage-price czars and the public proclamations that "physicians make too much money," these factors will assume greater proportion in the inflationary days that lie ahead.

More important by far is the fact that a legion of cost accountants lurking somewhere in the bowels of the Department of Health, Education, and Welfare will soon be wielding their budgetary axes on items of health care considered essential by the individual physician in the treatment of his patient. Individually the physician is powerless to resist this intrusion into his professional prerogatives, much less to defend himself against the charge that he is overutilizing for personal gain. Collectively, however, a union can at least have input through negotiation in defending the professional integrity of its members. Paradoxically, as this is always in the direction of broadening the scope of medical care, the physicians' unions find themselves in the unique position of being perhaps the most effective consumer advocates in the interest of their patients, the American public.

The old-line medical organizations have been powerless to impress upon insurance companies, hospital administration, and certainly government, the fact that physicians, once regarded as small businessmen-entrepreneurs, are no longer able to play a dominant role in the determination of their own professional lives or livelihoods. The quaintly archaic notion that a free marketplace still exists in medicine makes concerted action by physicians difficult to achieve. It is only when it is acknowledged that the triumvirate of our adversaries controls not only the quantity but the quality of the care we render, and the compensation we can hope to get for this, that we must move in the direction of demanding the same rights granted under labor law to any honest workmen, the right to bargain collectively in our own behalf and in that of our patients.

Government officials proclaim that health care is different from other goods and services—forgetting that food, clothing, and housing, industries of at least as basic necessity, are heavily unionized. No, we cannot be denied the rights of organized labor generally without bending the constitutional guarantees of equality.

The worry that unionization by doctors will strip them of their professional dignity and invite the imposition of even more controls is laughable. At this moment in history, when our profession is being nationalized, when we are being *selectively* socialized in a still-capitalistic society, talk about avoiding controls is specious. The punishment has actually preceded the crime.

Unions can accomplish many things, not the least of which is the stoppage of this long litany of strategic retreats and the increasingly defensive posture we have had to assume before the onslaught of our adversaries. By organizing early enough we can reasonably hope to control the development of health legislation, much as the Airline Pilots Association has had the dominant role in the development and regulation of legislation in their own industry. The "advisory commissions," whose advice is promptly ignored, may have satisfied the old-line medical organizations but they have no part in the future of the unions. They demand no less than collective bargaining, with access to mediation and arbitration of grievances. Unions will not only play a part in legislative advocacy but, as stated, in consumer advocacy.

Ultimately, if physicians are not to be reduced to a position of involuntary servitude, the right to withhold services is the last weapon they possess. This horrendous notion, that imperious and unfeeling physicians would leave patients torn, bleeding, and unattended, is sheer hogwash. Under all circumstances it can be safely assumed that no physician worthy of his degree would fail to render care to anyone in urgent need of that care. It can be stated, however, that physicians possess the power through concerted action to disrupt the comfort and convenience of any bureaucracy designed to control them, and that this can be easily done without denying anyone essential medical care. Physicians, with a longer history of dedicated service than politicians, simply cannot be manipulated into an acceptance of injuring or of rendering inferior care to their patients. Any blame for that must rest squarely with their adversaries. When it finally percolates into the politicians' consciousness that physicians are no longer meek and manipulable, all this talk about massive civil disobedience will become moot.

In these times of great change the opportunities at least equal the challenges. A proud and noble profession can only salvage both its pride and its nobility by its willingness to defend the principles it has come to represent. There are battles to be fought and spurs to be won, and they cannot be won by the faint-hearted, the complacent, or the self-seeking. The Era of Medical Unionism has begun!

Addendum by Samuel Wolfe, Guest Editor—It may be anticipated that unionization of the medical profession in the United States will increase sharply in the years ahead, especially when one considers that by the end of 1975 as many as 100,000 physicians, or close to 25 per cent, will be working primarily as salaried employees. While it is not easy to come by exact figures, some estimate that as many as 55,000 physicians in the United States already are affiliated with medical unions. At the national level, the American Federation of Physicians and Dentists, and the National Physicians Council, the latter affiliated with the American Federation of Labor-Congress of Industrial Organizations, are the principal bodies serving as national clearinghouses for activities in this field. While officially, the American Medical Association feels that both the professional and economic goals of the profession can be best achieved through programs of the AMA and its constituent societies across the country, it is clear that opposition to medical unionism by the AMA has diminished over the past 18 months. It is noteworthy that the AMA has recently reaffirmed the profession's tradition not to withhold medical services as a bargaining mechanism.

CHAPTER 6

Hospital Workers:
Class Conflicts In The Making

Barbara Ehrenreich and John H. Ehrenreich

In many of its characteristics, the hospital industry is distinct from other major American industries. For example, the product of the hospital industry is not a material commodity but a service which is viewed, in our society, as biologically necessary. The bulk of the industry operates on a "nonprofit" basis. The hospital work force is in many ways distinct from the industrial work force as a whole. It is a relatively highly skilled work force fragmented into a large and still growing number of job categories which are often legally defined. Within the hospital work force, the distinction between managerial and productive work is far less clear than it is in most industries. These and other peculiarities of the hospital industry have tended to obscure a class analysis of the hospital work force. In this article we attempt to locate the sources of class conflict within the hospital work force in the nature and organization of hospital work. Our analysis is based, in large measure, on formal interviews and informal discussions with hospital workers during the last five years.

Hospitals constitute one of the most rapidly growing and rapidly changing industries in the United States; a few decades ago they could hardly have been described as an "industry" at all. From the hospital workers' standpoint, the most obvious changes are in sheer size (from an average of 132 employees per short-term, nonfederal hospital in 1950 to 352 in 1972) and in the increased amount and complexity of equipment (from an average of $854,000 in assets per hospital in 1950 to $5,750,000 in 1972). Total short-term, nonfederal hospital employment tripled during the same period, from 662,000 in 1950 to 2,056,000 in 1972 (1, 2). And even these figures underestimate the qualitative significance of the change which has occurred in the urban centers since the figures include many rural hospitals which are still relatively small and technologically backward. Advances in the organization of health care occur first and are more concentrated in the big cities. There, the old neighborhood hospital has been all but replaced by, or swallowed up in, giant medical complexes, each containing thousands of beds, employing thousands of workers, and controlling assets which may run into the hundreds of millions.

The consolidation of the urban hospital industry into larger and larger units has been accompanied by basic changes in the functioning of hospitals. Most American hospitals are legally "nonprofit" but, encouraged by governmental and private "cost-plus" financing mechanisms and by government grants, many have become aggressively expansionist, rivalling "for-profit" corporations in their pursuit of growth in assets and

*Portions of this paper have appeared in *Monthly Review* (January 1973) and are reprinted by permission of the publisher.

revenues. With much justification, consumer groups have charged that many large urban medical centers are "not in business for people's health." Their priorities center around research, medical education, plant expansion, academic prestige, and high managerial salaries; patient care comes in virtually as a by-product (3).

Before the Second World War, and before the current hospital boom, the hospital work force was made up of doctors and trained nurses, plus a large group of unskilled, semidifferentiated workers. No segment of this work force could be considered in any sense analogous to industrial workers. The doctors and nurses were usually free-lancers or students, with no permanent attachment to the hospital. The others were economically marginal people, often handicapped, illiterate, or aged, who were paid barely enough for individual subsistence. With turnover rates for hospital workers in the range of 70 to 80 per cent per year, there was no body of American workers who could be said to comprise a stable hospital work force.

The explosive growth of the hospital industry in the last two decades has led to the formation of a hospital work force which is increasingly stable, highly differentiated, and in many other ways similar to the industrial work force. Semiskilled and unskilled hospital workers are no longer transients, or objects of charity, but long-term hospital employees who expect a day's wage for a day's work, and are increasingly turning to unions to make sure they get it. Skilled hospital workers, such as technicians and nurses, are now almost entirely full-time salaried employees. They, too, have been joining unions or pressing their professional associations into behavior that is increasingly union-like.

Skilled and unskilled hospital workers alike face working conditions which more and more resemble those in an industrial plant. There is an elaborate division of labor: One New York hospital lists 42 pay categories of service and maintenance workers (nurses' aides, porters, kitchen workers), 35 types of clerical workers (secretaries, ward clerks, medical-record librarians), and 38 varieties of technical and professional personnel (registered nurses, lab technicians, x-ray technicians, physical therapists). And even this understates the fragmentation, for a pay category such as "clinical lab technician" includes technicians specialized in hematology, cytology, and urinalysis. As in many industrial settings, workers in hospitals participate in an increasingly small part of the productive process—a situation which is conducive to the familiar industrial syndrome of work place alienation.

But despite this apparent "industrialization" of hospital workers, the hospital worker is not just an industrial worker whose product happens to be medical care. Hospital work is different from industrial work and the hospital worker faces contradictions which have only limited analogies in manufacturing industries or even in other service industries. First, and most obvious, is the fact that the central product of hospital work is not some artifact of questionable value, but a service whose value is self-evident. And no amount of automation or specialization can completely obscure this fact. No matter how fragmented or menial their jobs, no matter how bad their working conditions, hospital workers at all skill levels commonly express a degree of commitment to service, to doing one's best, that would be beyond the wildest dreams of an industrial personnel manager. A technician told us: "I personally like [working in a hospital] because you're doing something for people . . . I couldn't work eight hours a day with no real purpose." A nurses' aide said: "There is more in a job than bringing home a paycheck, and when I know that I've done something to help someone who couldn't help himself, that is my reward." And a ward clerk explaining why she put up with the frustrations of her job, told us: "You still have the patients. You do the best you can." (Indeed, hospital managements have often successfully exploited the workers' service ethic to avert strikes and unionization.)

But the hospital workers' service ethic does not guarantee a selfless devotion to the hospital as an institution. To the extent that the modern hospital is not a "mission of mercy," but a business enterprise whose management structure and priorities are not dissimilar from those of an industrial corporation, the service ethic is a potentially subversive force. "If you have any feelings of responsibility for the patients, you can't stand it any more," said one practical nurse. Another told us: "You have to see this place as a giant bureaucracy. I'm at the bottom of it, or maybe the patients are, and there's not a lot an individual can do." A nurses' aide who is a local union official at New York's Bellevue Hospital summed it up: "Some of our people feel they're not so much in the patient-care area as catering to the comfort of administrators.... They [the administration] say they want patient care but they don't make it possible."

The second major peculiarity of hospital work lies in the organization of work. For technologic and historical reasons hospital work features a high degree of functional interdependence between workers of extremely different rank within the hospital and extremely different social status outside it. For example, a surgical operation commonly requires the cooperative efforts of a team whose members range in rank from surgeon to aides. The surgeon has had eight or more years of postcollege training; he may earn more than $100,000 a year; he may sit on one of the hospital's key management committees, on the medical board, or even on the board of directors. The aide may have no high school education, earn less than $7,000, and lack even the authority to make a simple suggestion. But in the operation itself, they are both essential participants, as the aide can easily demonstrate by making a small but fatal mistake. There is thus a continual contradiction between the worker's sense of her of his own importance in the productive process and her or his total lack of importance in the institution.

To put it another way, there is a very real contradiction between the doctor's actual functional importance and his inflated status within the hospital. (Here we are not speaking of the doctors-in-training, the interns and residents, whose position is much more ambiguous.) As the division of hospital labor increases and the doctor delegates more and more of his historic functions to members of the nursing and technical staff, he becomes at least as dependent on the skills of other workers as they are on his. "You could imagine a hospital with no doctors. Everything would get done just the same," a nurse in a New York City municipal hospital told us. "But try to imagine a hospital with no nurses. It would be chaos. The patients would all die of neglect." Similarly, the technicians could argue that, without them, the doctor would be virtually unable to diagnose a single case.

The doctor's position has no parallel in industry. On the one hand, he is a top executive in the hospital "corporation." On the other hand, he is simply a highly skilled production worker, working side by side with nurses, aides, and technicians, and subject to their continual surveillance. They are the first, and usually the only, witnesses to his failures—unnecessary postoperative complications, prescriptions for the wrong dosages of drugs, faulty diagnoses, and so forth. And they are the harshest judges of his ethical standards: Does he discriminate against poor or nonwhite patients? Does he care more about whether he can publish the case than whether he can cure the patient? Insofar as he has become an integral part of hospital management, his individual shortcomings, however minor, serve to discredit the entire authority structure of the institution.

The difference between the doctor-manager and his coworkers is not just one of rank within the hospital, but of absolute social status. In fact, the hospital's elaborate and militaristic system of rank identifications—uniforms, pins, titles—is hardly necessary. Everyone knows that in the big city hospital, white males are likely to be doctors, white women to be nurses or technicians, nonwhites to be aides and janitors, and so on. Doctors are 98 per cent white, 93 per cent male, and predominantly from upper- and upper-middle-class families (4, 5). Nurses and technicians are usually lower-middle-class and white; 98 per cent of registered nurses, 96 per cent of practical nurses, and 70 per cent of technicians are women (6; 7, pp. 235, 238). Aides, cooks, and maids are lower-class men and women; in the big cities of the north, they are usually black, Chicano, or Puerto Rican. (In New York City's municipal hospitals, 80-90 per cent are nonwhite (8).)

This class, race, and sex stratification is due not so much to biased hiring practices, as to the fact that in the hospital virtually everyone remains at his or her entry-level job. Compared to other industries there is an almost complete lack of job mobility, even though there is often a great deal of functional interchangeability between the various types of workers. For example, practical nurses commonly possess the same skills as RNs (Registered Nurses) and are often assigned responsibilities theoretically and legally reserved for RNs (at no extra pay, of course). But the only way a practical nurse can gain the title, the status, and the pay of the RN is by attending school full-time for at least two years. So the practical nurse, like the aide below her and the RN above her, tends to remain where she started, i.e. at exactly the level toward which she was tracked long ago in public school.

The result is an occupational hierarchy which seems to have been almost designed to promote conflict. There is an unbridgeable gap—of both institutional rank and absolute social status—between the technical and managerial elite (doctors and administrators) and the great bulk of the work force. The structural inequity of this hierarchy is made inescapable by a productive process which mixes the two groups in intimate daily contact. Finally, there is a growing substantive antagonism between the two groups over the fundamental issue of the purpose of work: human service versus the hospital managers' corporate priorities.

To have meaningful work and to be adequately recognized for doing it, both materially and in terms of respect and status within the institution—these are the hospital workers' real and conscious needs. So what prevents the collective expression of these needs? What maintains the hospital hierarchy in the face of the contradictions we have described? There are two main stabilizing forces, operating in part on different sets of hospital workers. For the unskilled and semiskilled workers, there are forces which lead to a kind of passive alienation from the content of their work. For the skilled workers, there is the ideology of professionalism. The first denies the service ethic and accepts the class division within the hospital. The second denies the class division and diverts the service ethic into a professional "ethic" of institutional loyalty.

Undoubtedly many of the lower-level workers enter hospital work because they can find no other semiskilled jobs in the cities. But a large majority do start with the expectation that there is some special meaning and dignity to hospital work. Conditions (in even the "best" hospitals), however, are enough to undermine the efforts of even the most dedicated workers—understaffing, inadequate supplies and equipment, obstructive red tape, priorities given to non-patient-care functions. In their training or orientation, lower-level workers are warned against taking it all too seriously. "Do not try to achieve perfection in everything, because, admirable as it is, it is an invitation to failure and often is most impracticable," warns one text for practical nurses (9). Suggestions and innovations from the ranks are not encouraged, and are usually viewed as "trouble-making." A practical nurse told us: "The employee is not supposed to question anything. The supervisors will write up anything as 'insubordination'." And an aide told us, "You go to your supervisor [about a patient care problem]. She doesn't do anything. Eventually you stop caring, too." Again and again we heard the refrain, "After a while you just don't give a damn." You become the adjusted, "industrialized" worker, for whom hospital work is just a job.

The recent wave of hospital unionization has done much to reinforce the psychological industrialization of the lower-rank hospital workers. Like unions in other industries, hospital workers' unions do not challenge the nature of the "product" or the organization of work. Their interest in qualitative, service issues has been largely a matter of public relations rhetoric, and their efforts to reform the occupational hierarchy have been minimal. Leon Davis, President of New York's Local 1199 (which represents some 62,000 hospital workers in New York, New Jersey, and Connecticut), wrote in the union's magazine a response to an attempt at involving the union in efforts to change the structure and control of hospitals: "Our basic and primary responsibility is to achieve a degree of power in order to deal with wages, fringe benefits, job security, grievance machinery and dignity on the job" (10). To involve the union in issues such as the internal organization or priorities of hospitals would, Davis continued, be so divisive as to "tear this union apart." In effect, the union's message to the workers is, "We can't do anything about the fact that you have a meaningless dead-end job, but we can get you paid more for doing it." In fact, the hospitals pass wage hikes for hospital workers onto consumers, in the form of either higher charges or reduced services. So by concentrating on economic demands, without in any way challenging the hospital hierarchy and its non-service priorities, the unions implicitly place the needs of the workers in conflict with the needs of the consumer—the ultimate alienation.

Professionalism is a factor which is uniquely important in the hospital industry (though it is also present in a number of other "new working class' work settings) and deserves a much more careful examination. Some 40 per cent of all nonmanagerial hospital workers are in job categories which consider themselves "professional" (7, p. 73). There is no question but that the hospital work force is relatively highly skilled: what is peculiar is that virtually every technically trained category in the hospital has pretensions of professionalism. A technician working for a drug company, for instance, would probably not consider herself a professional; in a hospital, she would. This is not simply a matter of individual self-appraisal, either. X-Ray technicians, inhalation therapists, physical therapists, and a host of other job categories boast their own professional associations, complete with ethical codes, publications, conventions, dues, and so on.

Obviously, to make sense out of this rampant professionalism, it is necessary first to clear up what is meant by a "profession." The word calls to mind lengthy, specialized training, high standards of performance, ethics which transcend personal desires, and other worthy attributes. Doctors and lawyers come to mind. The importance of these images is not that they are accurate but that they reflect the special status accorded to professional workers in our society. They usually earn more and are almost always accorded more respect than other workers. But performing what whould generally be called "professional" duties in a "professional" manner does not suffice to make a worker a "professional." For example, a practical nurse and a registered nurse may perform exactly the same duties at an identical level of technical and ethical standards. But only the RN is a real professional, i.e. a licensed member of a legally recognized professional group.

Thus the word "professional" has two sets of meanings—one based in popular imagery and the other in legal reality. In the latter sense, a profession is an organized occupational group which has been granted a monopoly over the performance of certain functions and a certain degree of autonomy in carrying them out. For example, the medical profession has a legal monopoly over the prescribing of drugs, surgical practice, the classifying of people as fit or unfit for a variety of functions, and so forth. It has almost complete autonomy to police its members and to set standards for the admission of new members.

Once we have said that a profession is a legal entity, we have said that it is also a social and political entity. A group does not become a profession by winning a mass vote of confidence, but by winning the recognition of courts and legislatures. In the words of sociologist Eliot Freidson (11, p. 72):

> A profession attains and maintains its position by virtue of the protection and patronage of some elite segment of society which has been persuaded that there is some special value in its work. Its position is thus secured by the political and economic influence of the elite which sponsors it—an influence that drives competing occupations out of some areas of work, that discourages others by virtue of the competitive advantages conferred on the chosen occupation, and that requires still others to be subordinated to the profession.

The American medical profession provides one of the clearest examples. In the mid-19th century there was no American medical profession, only a welter of competing sects. The emergence of one group of doctors as the modern medical profession was due less to their technical superiority (they had little at that time) than to the conscious intervention of the upper class (and particularly of the Carnegie and Rockefeller Foundations) (12). (Today, of course, the medical profession is a political force in its own right, quite capable of defending its own interests without overt upper-class intervention.)

To return to the numerous other health professions: These have a much lower status than the medical profession. In fact, there is a definite hierarchy of health professions. At the top is the medical profession, the only completely autonomous health profession, the only one whose authority was derived directly from the upper class. All the other health professions were sanctioned by, and are to varying degrees supervised by, the medical profession itself. The ideologies of these professions reflect their subordinate status and create, in the professional worker, an internalized "sense of one's place."

Consider first the nursing profession. RNs occupy an intermediate position in the hospital hierarchy—subordinate to the doctors, but in a supervisory role with respect to practical nurses, aides, and (depending on the hospital) several other kinds of semiskilled workers. Ideologically, nursing professionalism combines the authoritarianism necessary for the nurse's supervisory role with the submissiveness implicit in her relation to the doctors. In a way, this sense of mixed status could be said to come "naturally" to nurses: RNs are women, usually from the lower-middle-class. Being women, they have been socialized to be subordinate to the male doctors. Being of high enough economic class to have afforded nursing education, they can easily feel superior to the aides and practical nurses.

This pattern goes back to the origins of the nursing profession in the late 19th century. Nursing as we know it was invented by a small number of upper-class reformers, largely under the intellectual leadership of Florence Nightingale. The Nightingale nurse was defined by her "character," rather than by her skills; and the nursing "character" was modeled after the upper-class Victorian lady: To the doctor, she brought the wifely virtue of absolute obedience; to the patient, she brought the selfless devotion of a mother; to the lower-level hospital employees she brought the firm but kindly discipline of a household manager, accustomed to handling servants. She desired none of the doctor's skills or prerogatives. His professionalism stemmed from the masculine realm of scientific thought, hers from a kind of innate feminine spirituality.

As far as hospital management is concerned, the historic professional self-image of the nurse is as serviceable today as it ever was. Nursing is still a "feminine" profession, and nurses are still trained to be "ladies" (i.e. to imitate the manners and style of upper-class women) and hence to feel a class above the workers they must supervise. Today, however, the four-year liberal arts degree is replacing "character" as the hallmark of class. If the nurses' professional organizations have their way, "professional" nursing, i.e. supervisory roles, will be restricted to the graduates of four-year, college-based nursing programs. There is still no threat to the doctor, because baccalaureate nursing education is no richer in scientific content than the old hospital training. All it takes is a smattering of high-priced liberal arts courses to make sure that the nurse is a class above her subordinates.

The other submedical hospital workers' professions are narrower and more craft-oriented than the nursing and medical professions. Each comprises a narrow set of functions spun off by the medical profession in the last 30 years or so—medical technology, inhalation therapy, physical therapy, and so forth. Organizationally, these relatively new "allied" health professions lack even the dubious independence of the nursing profession. For example, accreditation of schools for training allied health workers is controlled by the American Medical Association Council on Medical Education. Certification of individuals in most occupations is jointly supervised by the allied professional society and its parent medical-specialty society (for example, the American College of Radiologists in the case of x-ray technicians).

The creation of the allied health professions represents a kind of pact between highly unequal parties. The medical profession delegates one of its functions and agrees to recognize the new practitioners as fellow "professionals." (Presumably there is no physician's task so inconsequential as to be entrusted to nonprofessionals.) In practice this means that doctors and hospitals agree to give preference in hiring to certified members of the new occupational grouping, or at least to pay them more than uncertified persons who may have simply acquired the skill in question. Members of the new allied health profession, in turn, agree to "keep in their place": to submit to medical domination of accreditation and certification, to confine their work activities within limits set by physicians, and so forth.

The ideology of the allied health professions is amply illustrated by this credo of the medical technologist:

> As a medical technologist, I am proud, with a pride that is tinctured with a true humility, with a pride in being one of the trio in the medical profession, the physician, the nurse, and the medical technologist, each of whom functions in his distinct way. As a medical technologist, I am independent, with a cooperative spirit in working with my fellows in the medical profession. I do not want to encroach upon anyone else's premises. (From *The American Journal of Medical Technology*, cited in reference 11, p. 68.)

To the hospital, the nurses and the new allied professionals are in a sense workers who do not see themselves as workers, who do not look on their work as merely a job. In the words of one typical textbook for nursing students, the distinguishing characteristic of a *professional* nurse is that:

> . . . her primary source of personal satisfaction comes from her knowledge of service rendered rather than from material rewards. . . . She sees nursing not as just a job but as a lifetime career of human service. . . . She doesn't just work at nursing, she *is* a nurse—a professional nurse (13).

The advantages of this attitude to the hospital are obvious: *Workers* are too quickly alienated by fragmented jobs; true *professionals* rejoice in the exercise of their craft. *Workers* identify with other workers in their institution, and can unite on the spot around common grievances. *Professionals* identify only with other members of their profession, and look to a distant professional society for long-term advancement. Finally, *workers* need discipline and close supervision; the true *professional* can be trusted to adhere to the ethics and standards of his profession in any situation.

Conditions of work in the modern industrialized hospital engender a uniquely clear set of class and caste antagonisms. The hospital joins, in the intimacy of its productive processes, members of the upper and upper-middle classes, whose institutional functions are increasingly managerial, with a large body of workers from less privileged strata of society—women, the poor and near-poor, and, in certain localities, nonwhites. It pits these two groups—the managerial elite and the rest of the work force—against each other in conflicts, not all of which can be resolved without a radical recasting of the nature and purpose of hospital work. There is the classic industrial conflict over wages and working conditions, the improvement of which necessarily threatens management spending priorities. There is the worker's need for meaningful, service-oriented jobs, which necessarily threatens management priorities for the hospital as a business enterprise; there is the worker's need for advancement in skills and for participation as a real "team" member—needs which run headlong into the doctors' defensive monopoly over the scientific underpinnings of the production process.

But, as we have seen, there are forces at work which serve both to obscure these needs and to prevent collective action around them. Lower-level workers are encouraged by management and by their unions to set aside qualitative demands in return for economic gains. Skilled workers are seduced by the ideology of professionalism into foregoing both qualitative and quantitative satisfactions in return for an abstract sense of status. The result is an increasing division of the nonmanagerial hospital work force into two groups with opposing class identifications: on the one hand, a proletarianized body of unskilled and semiskilled workers, and, on the other hand, an equally large group of skilled workers who, through the device of professionalism, are allowed to participate—however vicariously—in the very real status of the doctors.

REFERENCES

1. *Hospitals (J.A.H.A.), Guide Issue*, August 1, 1971.
2. American Hospital Association. *Hospital Statistics*, 1973.
3. Health Policy Advisory Center. *The American Health Empire: Power, Profits and Politics*, Ch. 1-5. Random House, New York, 1970.
4. U.S. Bureau of the Census. *Statistical Abstract of the United States, 1972*, p. 69. U.S. Government Printing Office, Washington, D.C., 1972.
5. Fein, R., and Weber, G. *The Financing of Medical Education*, pp. 101-107. McGraw-Hill, New York, 1971.

6. U.S. Department of Labor. *Handbook on Women Workers,* p. 96. U.S. Government Printing Office, Washington, D.C., 1969.
7. U.S. Bureau of the Census. *Statistical Abstract of the United States, 1973.* U.S. Government Printing Office, Washington, D.C., 1973.
8. Gilpatrick, E. *The Occupational Structure of New York City Hospitals,* Vol. I, Health Services Mobility Study. Research Foundation, City University of New York, New York, 1968.
9. Ross, C. F. *Personal and Vocational Relationships in Practical Nursing,* Ed. 3, p. 103. Lippincott, Philadelphia, 1969.
10. Local 1199, Drug and Hospital Union, Retail, Wholesale, and Department Store Union (AFL-CIO). *Drug and Hospital News,* December 1969.
11. Freidson, E. *The Profession of Medicine.* Dodd, Mead, New York, 1970.
12. Stevens, R. *American Medicine and the Public Interest,* pp. 55-74. Yale University Press, New Haven, 1971.
13. Kelly, C. W. *Dimensions of Professional Nursing,* Ed. 2, pp. 15-16. Macmillan, New York, 1968.

CHAPTER 7

An International Perspective On Strikes And Strike Threats By Physicians: The Case of Chile

Roberto Belmar and Victor W. Sidel

A strike is still usually thought of as a weapon employed by workers—viewed as those who are relatively deprived and powerless and have no other means of redress—against those who exploit them. The Chilean doctors' strikes of 1972-1973 had far different antecedents and purposes, and in these seemed to differ from other doctors' strikes as well (1). In this article we attempt to analyze critically the causes, development, and results of the Chilean doctors' strikes.

THE ALLENDE HEALTH PROGRAM

In September 1970 the candidate of the Unidad Popular, a coalition of parties of the left, won the presidential election of Chile with a plurality of 36.3 per cent of the popular vote (2). Dr. Salvador Allende Gossens, a physician, thus became the first self-proclaimed socialist democratically elected to the presidency of a nonsocialist nation in the Western Hemisphere. He rapidly developed a strong new social and economic policy for Chile. This policy was characterized by the nationalization of mining industries, especially those for copper, iron, and coal, and of selected other basic industries and of banking; redistribution of the land of the *latifundios* (huge farms) to those who worked the land; changes in income patterns in favor of previously lesser-paid workers; reopening full-time of industries closed or functioning only part-time because of the severe recession during the previous administrations; and reorientation of production priorities toward the specific needs of poorer people (3, 4).

In addition to the new economic policies there was a strong movement to strengthen programs for the provision of human services. In health, this was initiated through the Plan Sexenal de Salud (Six-Year Health Plan) (5). This plan had as one of its basic goals the incorporation of community organizations into health decision making through the "democratization" of the Servicio Nacional de Salud (SNS), the national health service of Chile (6). The SNS, which had provided medical care for Chile's blue-collar workers and for its poor (70 per cent of the Chilean population) as well as prevention and environmental protection services for all of Chile's people since 1952 (7), was also to be strengthened by delegation of greater powers in health planning, decentralization and elimination of excess bureaucracy, introduction of new models of ambulatory care, and improvement in programs such as those for prevention and treatment of alcoholism and for milk distribution. These programs have also been described in English by Navarro (8) and by Waitzkin and Modell (9, 10).

Community Participation

The incorporation of the community into health decision-making processes became the policy of the SNS under President Allende. This policy was officially stated in Decreto Numero 602, issued in August 1971 shortly after Allende took office, which directed the creation in every health center of a "local health council" (11). This council was to include members elected by the local community organizations as well as representatives of the local branch of the Colegio Medico (the Chilean Medical Association, to which all doctors were required to belong in order to practice medicine), of the nonphysicians' Professional Personnel Association, and of the "nonprofessionals' " Health Workers Union. (These groups are described in greater detail later in this paper.)

During the three years of the Allende administration the process of democratization of the SNS appeared to be developing successfully. At least 400 local health councils were established. Local community members for the first time began to have a real role in discussions of local health matters and in decisions on the use of scarce health resources. The developing roles of the local health councils included the training of community volunteers in the prevention of alcoholism and of communicable disease and the creation of new satellite neighborhood health centers (12, 13).

Health Planning

The process of definition of health care needs and goals, planning for the optimal use of resources, organization and administration of programs, and program evaluation was to be nationally coordinated but locally implemented (14). For this purpose there was established a national planning office to advise the local health councils and the local health officials on the process of health planning; to provide norms for the following year's planning process, including the expected output for every health resource; to coordinate the budget of the entire SNS; and to initiate a national process of evaluation of the different programs (15).

One of the important changes in health planning was the clear definition of three different kinds of programs—those related to people, environment, and sociocultural development (16). Some of the programs related to the people were the Child Health Program, the Adolescent Health Program, and the Health Program for the Aged (17). Many of these programs had subprograms for specific problems such as prevention and treatment of malnutrition and venereal disease, early detection of cervical cancer, and family planning. The programs related to environment included Environmental Sanitation, Occupational Medicine, Food Hygiene Control, and Zoonosis Control. The programs related to sociocultural development included the Democratization of the SNS (discussed above) and the Mental Health Program, including its alcoholism control subprogram.

The planning office sponsored conferences and seminars, distributed informational materials, and used every possible means of communication to involve community members in this work. The health workers and community members were encouraged to help define the goals, the methods, the cost, and the evaluation techniques for each program. There was thus an attempt to achieve an integrated process of health planning in which important decisions were made through the interaction among the health workers, the health center, and the members of the community itself (9).

Teams of health workers in the health centers had responsibilities in all of the programs and therefore helped to integrate them at the local level. The programs helped ensure that local health workers emphasize preventive rather than therapeutic efforts.

Decentralization and Reduction of Bureaucracy

Success in the two preceding efforts required that the local health workers and the local community have sufficient freedom of action in planning and administration. For this reason the SNS gave the director of each health center power to manage the personnel and the budget of his center with the advice of the local health council.

Ambulatory Medical Care

The Six-Year Health Plan encouraged the development of local health centers and satellite clinics. They were to provide 24-hour medical services all year round. Each center was to develop the concept of differentiated levels of medical care, in which each member of the health team was to deal with health problems specific to his or her level of training (9, 18-21). The levels of personnel to be used were volunteers, medical students, nurses, general practitioners, specialists, and subspecialists. Every health team had health workers who performed functions at each level of medical care. Each team had an assigned population to serve. In other words, there was an attempt to correlate the demands for service with the capacity of each member of the health team, similar in some ways to progressive care in the modern hospital.

One of the most outstanding new roles was that for students of medicine. They worked in the health centers during the last years of their medical studies. Their responsibilities included treating the most prevalent acute and chronic diseases in the population; educating adults on the process of medical care; developing groups for control of problems such as diabetes, hypertension, tuberculosis, alcoholism, and malnutrition; providing first aid for accidents at home and at work; setting up and staffing a basic laboratory in the health center; and participating in the training of health volunteers (22, 23).

This new approach to ambulatory medical care was especially emphasized in the large urban areas such as those of Santiago and Concepcion. The Fifth Health Zone of the SNS (covering the city of Santiago) had 83 health centers, most in the poor sections of the city, providing free services to those covered by the National Health Service. Thirty centers were open 24 hours a day, 7 days a week, and another 25 were open from 8 a.m. to 10 or 12 p.m. This program provided services to about 2,000,000 people. This increase of care to the more deprived neighborhoods of the urban areas meant that the previous lengthy waits and de facto rejections from care in the ambulatory services were largely eliminated (24).

Special Subprograms

A number of new or expanded programs were developed as part of each health center. These included:

Anti-Alcoholism Campaign. Alcoholism is a highly prevalent health problem in Chilean society. Prevention was given an important role; volunteers were trained to educate the high-risk groups to avoid alcohol and to avoid social situations which induce people to drink. They were also trained to treat alcoholic patients who requested it with a new electric adversive technique based on feedback conditioning. In addition, many anti-alcoholism groups run by recovered alcoholics were initiated. This activity created for the first time a comprehensive care and prevention program for alcoholism and its medical and psychologic complications.

Milk Distribution Program. A milk program had been initiated under previous administrations but was vastly expanded during the Allende period. All children under 14 years of age received 500 ml of milk per day and children under 2 received enough milk for a full feeding schedule. As important in some ways as the milk itself was the education of mothers through the relationship developed with the health center as a result of this program (24, 25).

Results

The new health programs and the improved quality of life of the Chilean people—including redistribution of income and new housing—even over only 3 years produced some quantifiable results which demonstrate its impact. Changes in mortality rates and life expectancy from 1969 to 1972 are shown in Table 1.

Table 1

Health indices for Santiago and for all Chile, 1969-1972[a]

Health Indices	Chile		Santiago	
	1969	1972	1969	1972
Mortality rate for infant diarrhea per 1000 live births	15.6 (1968)	10.7	19.4	10.2
Infant mortality rate per 1000 live births	78.8	70.0 (65.3 in 1973)	55.0	48.8
Maternal mortality rate per 1000 live births	1.8	1.6 (1.3 in 1973)	1.4	1.2
Life expectancy at birth for males in years	58 (1967)	64	—	—

[a] Sources, references 26-32.

ORGANIZATIONS OF HEALTH WORKERS IN CHILE

An understanding of the impact of the changes in the Chilean SNS and their consequences requires an understanding of the other parts of the medical care system of

Chile. As noted above, the SNS covered about 70 per cent of the Chilean population for medical care services and 100 per cent of the population for preventive and environmental services (7, 33, 34). Twenty per cent of the population was covered by a fee-for-service program called SERMENA (Servicio Nacional de Empleados) initiated in 1968 (34, 35). This program served Chile's white-collar workers, who paid their fees to the physician with a payment voucher given to them by SERMENA. This order cost the patient only a third of its cash value to the doctor, the other two-thirds being provided from the insurance premiums paid by the employers and from general revenue funds. This system permitted the free selection of doctors and therefore was strongly supported by those in private practice; the method of payment also permitted local abuse, with some doctors demanding two or three payment vouchers from the patient for a single visit. The other 10 per cent of the Chilean population was covered entirely through fee-for-service payments by the patient to private practitioners (34).

The organizations for health workers in Chile were also very important in the functioning of health services. They included:

- *Colegio Medico*—This organization for physicians, which is known in the United States as the Chilean Medical Association, was a nongovernmental organization, but Chilean law required that all Chilean physicians had to be enrolled in order to practice medicine (36). For this reason it had quasi-governmental status and *was forbidden by law to organize a strike or otherwise interfere with health services* (36, 37).
- *Professional Personnel Association*—The Asociacion de Profesionales de la Salud was also nongovernmental and included dentists, nurses, midwives, and other health professionals.
- *National Federation of Health Workers*—The nonprofessional workers in the health centers and hospitals belonged to the Federacion Nacional de Trabajadores de la Salud (FENATS) which had 48,000 members.

Only 5 per cent of Chile's doctors worked full-time in the SNS, but an additional 80 per cent were employed part-time; the average work load for the part-time doctors was 4 hours a day. Almost all of the part-time doctors, and the 15 per cent of Chile's doctors who were not employed by the SNS, engaged in private practice (7).

RESPONSE OF THE COLEGIO MEDICO
TO THE ALLENDE ADMINISTRATION

The changes in the SNS under Allende increased the socialization of Chilean medicine in that increased services were provided to the population without charge at the time of service. This process reduced private practice not because the government was directly attacking the private doctors but because most people preferred to get the care offered by the SNS rather than the care provided by the private physicians (24). The real income of physicians in private practice therefore began to fall and the doctors, most of whom were members of the upper or upper middle class before they entered medical school, felt jeopardized by the socialist process as a whole and specifically by the decline in their income (38). Many of them had taken a clear political position against Allende after his election (39).

The actions taken by the Colegio Medico during the Allende government can be analyzed in three periods.

First Period: September 4, 1970-October 8, 1972

This period starts from the day Allende was elected president. The various professional organizations of Chile—those of the lawyers, engineers, architects, the Professional Personnel Association, the Colegio Medico, and others—initiated a process of negotiation with the government in an attempt to ensure that the basic structure of the society was maintained with only some superficial reforms. In the beginning of this period there was a friendly approach to the government by the Colegio Medico; they even presented a decoration to President Allende for his outstanding previous work in the field of public health (40).

Once the government started, however, to implement the policy of community participation in health and the policy of nationalization of the basic resources of the country, the professional associations and especially the Colegio Medico began to resist these changes, although still professing agreement with the goals of the administration. For example, there was consistent opposition to the formation of the local health councils (39). The community organizations, FENATS, and the Professional Personnel Association elected their representatives to the respective health councils in the health centers or in the hospitals, but the physician representatives were selected by a very slow process in a few cases and not at all in most cases. The reason given by the Colegio Medico and its local chapters was that Decreto Numero 602, which had established the councils, still needed explanatory regulations.

Meanwhile the Colegio Medico requested a large increase in the salaries of physicians paid by the SNS and in the payments through SERMENA. The government agreed to increase stipends for the year 1971-1972 for that portion of the doctors' time spent working in the public sector. In spite of this, the medical profession was very disturbed because they would have preferred an increase in the controlled fee-for-service fees.

During this initial period the Colegio Medico did not strike but improved its organization, created strong affiliations with the Professional Personnel Association (but not with FENATS), and tried to slow down the implementation of the new health policy.

One important issue during this period was the migration of physicians out of the country. Some doctors who disliked the new health policy but who were not prepared to fight it directly decided simply to leave the country. Although the seven-year education of each physician is estimated to cost Chilean society $20,000 (in Chile all medical education is free to the student), the government did not put any barriers in the way of those who wanted to leave. Approximately 350 doctors (6 per cent) of a total of 5,572 active physicians left Chile during this period (41). This migration, and the limited time that the remaining doctors spent in NHS work, increased the needs of the NHS for additional physician time. For this reason the government asked the Colegio Medico to certify for practice a number of physicians coming from Argentina, Uruguay, and Spain. The physicians from Spain, for example, had been carefully selected by examination by recruiters there (42). The Colegio Medico used all its resources to stop the entrance of the foreign doctors, especially the group coming from Spain. Thus during this first period there were significant policy differences between the SNS and the Allende administration but no open confrontation.

Second Period: October 8, 1972-March 1973

This period started with the first nationwide strike against the Allende government. All the organizations which opposed the government unified their forces in a so-called

"Democratic Front" and tried to destroy the administration through a national strike (43). This process started with the strike of the owners of trucks who, with their economic power jeopardized by the development of a governmental fleet of trucks, attempted to paralyze the economy with their strike. This was possible because Chile, a country 2660 miles in length, required the transportation of basic materials, food, and equipment by road to keep production going and to provide needed supplies. The Colegio Medico decided to back the actions of the truck owners by calling for a sympathy strike among physicians despite the fact that this was expressly forbidden by Chilean law. The reason for the strike was officially given as support for the strengthening of health services, but its timing left little doubt that it was political in nature. The strike order by the Colegio Medico was obeyed by about 65 per cent of the doctors. In addition, some of the other health workers joined the strike, but in far fewer numbers than did the doctors.

During this strike a process crucial to the maintenance of the health system was organized. The health councils, the other professional health workers, and the nonprofessional health workers not only largely did not support the strike, but they realized that they had to look for other kinds of medical care models in which doctors were not so indispensible. Many community volunteers and medical students joined the 35 per cent of physicians and the other health workers who kept the hospitals and health centers functioning. A new health movement was therefore begun which not only was an important factor in ending the doctor strike, but was also the starting point for further polarization of the two groups in the health field. Those who kept working stressed a new kind of medicine in which the community and its leaders, volunteers, and senior medical students performed increasingly important tasks in the SNS ambulatory care program. In Santiago alone there were 495 medical students working in this program. The group which continued working during the strike also emphasized prevention and health maintenance and the relationship of health to other parts of the social change process such as food distribution, housing, and integration with the work of the labor unions (44).

Because the health care system was able to continue to function without them, the doctors ended their strike before the March 1973 election. This election was critical in determining the future of the Allende administration reforms, and the opposition used all the means at its disposal—both legal and illegal, including boycotts and slowdowns—to attempt to destroy the popular backing of the government. The health field was no exception. Among the methods used were: (a) The key positions in local and regional health administration were still held by opposition doctors and from this vantage point they slowed down all the processes of administration, e.g. by failure to recognize the health councils or by distortion of the orders coming from the central administration. When the government tried to replace a few of those doctors, using legal procedures, the Colegio Medico started local strikes or further slowdown methods by their followers. (b) Local boycotts of the care of patients were conducted by having physicians work fewer hours in the SNS than their contracted time called for. When the administration tried to impose time-clock control, the local chapter of the Colegio Medico urged disobeying the law and refusal to use the time clock. Since the government was attempting to keep the situation peaceful, local health authorities were advised not to reduce salaries as a result of the absence of physicians and not to initiate investigations into the actions of the doctors. (c) The Colegio Medico changed its regulations to impose on its members the duty to obey a decision by the Colegio to strike, under the penalty of losing their licenses to practice medicine if they refused to strike.

Third Period: March 1973-September 11, 1973

This period started with the parliamentary election, in which 44.7 per cent of the voters backed the Unidad Popular (UP) (up from 36.3 per cent two years before), which was seen as a defeat for the Allende opposition (45). This was especially true because the election showed a maintenance of the support for the UP among the older and middle-age electors and a sharp increase in support among the young. If the trend were continued until presidential elections in September 1976, the UP would conceivably gain an absolute majority.

All the strikes, national and local, the slowdowns and boycotts, and the public denunciation of the government by the Colegio Medico reached their climax in the medical strike of August 1973. Again this strike was held in conjunction with a strike by truck owners and by other professional organizations. During this last strike, the Colegio Medico demanded the resignation of the president. There was little pretense that the strike was conducted for reasons related to medical care or even the immediate economic interests of the physicians. The clear political nature of the strike by the Colegio Medico against the Allende government was demonstrated by its statement:

> The marxist tenets sponsored and supported by your administration are drawing individuals, associations, guilds and groups of all kinds to the ranks in the lowering political struggle and, furthermore contribute to the involvement in politics at the national level of physicians and even the Medical Association itself . . . (46).

The Colegio's document continues with an analysis of the Chilean situation in which nine of ten of the points are related to day-to-day political events rather than medical issues. The document concludes with the following paragraph:

> Given the foregoing and being absolutely certain that the time is long past for changes that would have assured a lawful course for the Ship of State and a strict adherence to the Constitution and the Laws contained therein, a legitimate right of all citizens of Chile, we deem that the time has come to declare, publicly, patriotically and openly that, as colleagues of yours, Mr. President, we repudiate your Administration's handling of the Executive Branch and demand immediate redress (46).

When that "redress" did not come, the Colegio Medico sent another document to the president which concluded with this paragraph:

> In the past we have asked you to change your course . . . and to respect the Constitution and its laws, but until now you have not demonstrated your intention to do so. Therefore, we believe the time has come to ask you, as a patriotic and sincere gesture, to resign from your position as President of the Republic (47).

The strikes in which the Colegio Medico and its followers participated appeared to be an important factor in the initiation of the military coup which overthrew President Allende's government and led to his death on September 11, 1973.

DISCUSSION

The strike by the Colegio Medico and its followers against the Allende government had well-defined antecedents which can be discussed under four headings: community participation, change in the model for delivery of medical care, change in the status of the physician in Chilean society, and the political position of the leadership of the Colegio

Medico which had joined together with other forces in an attempt to overthrow the government.

Community Participation

As we have described, the SNS developed a system, clearly legal, to provide ways for community organizations and other health worker groups to share with doctors the responsibility for defining health policy in the health centers and hospitals. This process was criticized by the Colegio Medico as political interference in professional matters, especially when the health councils attempted to increase priorities for ambulatory care and preventive measures over those for hospital care. The process of socialization in Chile and community participation speeded the redistribution of resources from hospitals to health centers, the training of volunteers in medical work, the participation of health workers in other activities such as food distribution, transportation, local security and industrial production, and the demand for increasing the power of the community in the health decision-making process. The medical profession felt that its ability to control the health system decreased as the people's control increased.

Change in the Model for Delivery of Medical Care

The second element which helps to explain the opposition of the Colegio Medico to the Allende government was the new model of care, which stressed prevention, ambulatory care, joint planning of health programs and the work of health teams, and the development of differentiated levels of medical care. Since this approach was being institutionalized in the SNS, it appeared to work to the detriment of the doctors in private practice. This was understandable because 90 per cent of the doctors working in the SNS received the most important part of their income from private practice and even used the equipment of the hospitals of the SNS for their private practice patients, who largely came from the upper and upper middle classes. It is important to stress the point that the government did not attempt directly to eliminate or curtail private practice. The improved quality of the care provided by the SNS, the possibility of the white-collar workers covered by SERMENA being voluntarily incorporated into SNS, and the social orientation of the new generation of medical students appeared to jeopardize the traditional private practice values of the medical profession. The Colegio Medico felt that the new policy portended a complete socialization of the health care resources of Chile into a unified national health service.

Change in Status of the Physician

The physician in Chile had previously held the highest rank in prestige among all the professions and occupations in the country, higher than senators, judges, high-ranking military officers, priests, or bankers. The Colegio Medico believed that community participation, the democratization of the health system, and the health team approach would lower the prestige of the physician in society. This was clearly demonstrated by the conclusion of an advertisement published by the junta in the *New York Times* in February 1974 in response to one published by the Emergency Committee to Save Chilean Health Workers: ". . . Allende was planning a state medical system whereby doctors would lose their professional status" (48).

Leadership of the Colegio Medico in the Opposition Movement

A final important reason why the doctors struck was the leading role played by the Colegio Medico's leaders in the political movement in Chile. Frank political statements against the government were made not only in relation to health policy, but in relation to all the aspects of social change. The opposition of the Colegio to President Allende in part expressed the alliance of the Colegio with upper-class forces which perceived the new model of society in Chile as a threat to their status and income.

The relationship of the Colegio Medico, and therefore of the doctors' strikes, to the opposition seeking the overthrow of the legally elected government of Chile was further seen in the acts of the Colegio Medico following the coup and the assumption of power by a military junta. The Colegio, despite its own Code of Ethics which calls for it to protest and defend physicians in jeopardy (49), actually collaborated in the selection of physicians and other health workers for imprisonment and acquiesced by silence in their torture and execution (50). The secretary general of the Colegio Medico has acknowledged that physicians supporting the junta have participated in denunciation of physicians who supported the Allende health care system (9, 51) and particularly of physicians who opposed the doctors' strikes (9). The military junta health authorities actually occupied offices for a time directly in the headquarters of the Colegio.

CONCLUSIONS

It seems clear that the Chilean doctors' strikes were only in part related to economic protection of the doctors and even less to the strengthening of health services, the usually stated reasons for doctors' strikes. The strikes were, for the most part, clearly political in nature.

There are those who assert that medicine can and should be apolitical and that both the Chilean physicians who supported the Allende health program and those who helped to destroy it are equally at fault (49). With this we profoundly disagree. Medicine, if it is to provide the best care for all people, must in part be political, not in the sense of political influences in the care of the individual patient but in the sense that the establishment and maintenance of optimal or even adequate health services must be part of a political process that involves all people and all services in the society. The issue here is not that doctors worked along political lines, but the methods chosen to do it. One group—those who supported the Allende changes—worked to organize communities and to broaden and strengthen health services for those who needed them most. The other group—represented by the Colegio Medico—used clearly illegal means both before and after the coup for political ends to diminish and even to destroy health services and those who attempted to provide them. In this they, in our view, overstepped the bounds of acceptable action for physicians—and for any citizen for that matter—and engaged in criminal acts. There may indeed be times when doctors' strikes are justifiable on either humane or economic grounds; Chile's examples are not among them.

REFERENCES

1. Badgley, R. F., and Wolfe, S. *Doctors' Strike: Medical Care and Conflict in Saskatchewan.* Atherton Press, New York, 1967; Macmillan Company, Toronto, 1967 and 1971.
2. Feinberg, R. E. *The Triumph of Allende: Chile's Legal Revolution.* Mentor Books, New York, 1972.
3. Petras, J. Chile after Allende: A tale of three coups. *Monthly Review* 21: 12-20, December 1973.

4. Steenland, K. Two years of popular unity in Chile: Balance sheet. *New Left Review* 78: 1-25, March-April 1973.
5. *Plan Sexenal de Salud.* Servicio Nacional de Salud de Chile, Chile, 1970.
6. Zimbalist, A. Worker's control: Its structure under Allende. *Monthly Review* 3: 39-42, March 1974.
7. Hall, T. L., and Díaz, S. Social security and health care patterns in Chile. *Int. J. Health Serv.* 1(4): 362-377, 1971.
8. Navarro, V. What does Chile mean? *Health and Society* 93-130, Spring 1974.
9. Waitzkin, H., and Modell, H. Medicine, socialism and totalitarism: Lessons from Chile. *New Engl. J. Med.* 291: 171-177, 1974.
10. Modell, H., and Waitzkin, H. Medicine and socialism in Chile. *Berkeley Journal of Sociology*, in press.
11. *Decreto 602.* Servicio Nacional de Salud, Chile, August 30, 1971.
12. *Programa de Desarrollo Socio Cultural.* Direccion General Servicio Nacional de Salud, Chile, 1972.
13. Aldunate, A. Participacion y actitud de las poblaciones ante organizaciones poblacionales. Flacso University of Chile, 1973.
14. Ahumada, J., et al. *Programacion de la Salud.* Scientific Publication of the Pan American Health Organization, Washington, D.C.. 1965.
15. Sepulveda, C., et al. *Tendencias actuales de la planificacion. Chile Cuadernos Medico Sociales* 12: 22-33, 1972.
16. *Plan operativo para la organizacian de las servicios de Salud.* Direccion General Servicio Nacional de Salud, Chile, 1972.
17. *Modelo de Programacion, 1972.* Oficina de Planificacion Servicio Nacional de Salud, Chile, 1971.
18. *Programa de Atencion Medica Externa.* V Zona de Salud, Servicio Nacional de Salud, Chile, 1972.
19. Requena, M. Programa de Atencion Medica Ambulatoria en el SNS. Direccion General de Salud, Chile, November 1971.
20. Belmar, R., and Sidel, V. W. A new approach to ambulatory care: The Chilean experience. *Clinical Research 22*: 376, 1974.
21. *Niveles de Atencion Medica en la A.M.E.* V Zona de Salud, Servicio Nacional de Salud, Chile, 1973.
22. Belmar, R., et al. Teaching of public health and social medicine. *Rev. Medica de Chile*, April 1971.
23. *Funciones del Auxiliar Tecnico.* V Zona de Salud, Decreto Circular 2341, SNS, Chile, June 25, 1973.
24. Kandell, J. Chile's poor get more medical aid. *New York Times*, March 31, 1973.
25. Belnap, D. E. Chile maps plans to get citizens to drink milk. *Los Angeles Times*, March 15, 1971.
26. Urrutia, F. *Servicio Nacional de Salud, Situacion actual y perspectivas.* SNS Document, Chile, December 1968.
27. Rosselot, J. Maternal and child health in Latin America. *Bol. Of. Sanit. Panam.* 6: 21-33, 1972.
28. Annual Report of V Health Zone, SNS, Chile, 1970.
29. Annual Report of V Health Zone, SNS, Chile, 1972.
30. Population Data. Department of Statistics, National Health Service, Chile, 1973.
31. *United Nations Demographic Yearbook*, 1970.
32. *Defunciones.* Department of Statistics, NHS, Chile, 1968, 1969, 1970, 1971 and 1972.
33. Hall, T. L. Chile health manpower study: Methods and problems. *Int. J. Health Serv.* 1(2): 166-184, 1971.
34. Juricic, B. Algunas consideraciones sobre Gastos en Salud en Chile, su financiamiento. *Chile Cuadernos Medico Sociales* 3: 17-22, 1973.
35. *Ley 16781* de Medicina Curativa. Republica de Chile, Chile, 1968.
36. *Ley 9263.* Republica de Chile, Chile, 1948.
37. *Estatuto Administrativo de la Republica de Chile.* Republica de Chile, undated.
38. Jegtanovic, P. *Estudio sobre Determinociones del Arancel del Colegio.* Communication of the Department of Public Health of the Colegio Medico de Chile, 1973.
39. Alvayay, J. Iterinanio de la columnia y la violencia Chile. *Boletin Colegio Medico de Valparaiso*, March 1973.
40. Vida Medica. Colegio Medico, Chile, 1971.
41. *El Mercurio.* Deficit Medico, Chile, May 12, 1974.
42. Belmar, R. Questionnaires for selection of foreign doctors. Direccion General SNS, Chile, 1972.
43. Argus, A. Medicine and politics in Chile. *World Medicine* 9: 15-44, April 1974.
44. Zimbalist, A., and Stalling, B. Showdown in Chile. *Monthly Review* 25: 1-25, October 1973.
45. Garcia, M. G. The death of Salvador Allende. *Harper's Magazine*, p. 11, May 1974.
46. Open letter to the President of the Republic. Colegio Medico de Chile, August 1973.
47. El Colegio Medico to the President of the Republic. Colegio Medico de Chile, August 26, 1973.
48. Junta Embassy of Chile in U.S. The real history of the persecution of doctors in Chile. An answer to the Emergency Committee to Save Chilean Health Workers. *New York Times*, February 10, 1974.

49. Jonsen, A. R., Paredes, A., and Sagan, L. Doctors in politics: A lesson from Chile. *New Engl. J. Med.* 291: 472-473, 1974.
50. Report of the Chicago Commission of Inquiry into the Status of Human Rights in Chile, Chicago, 1974.
51. Kandell, J. Thirteen doctors in Chile reported slain after the coup. *New York Times*, April 8, 1974.

CHAPTER 8

Unions and Strikes In The National Health Service In Britain

David Widgery

Over the past five years in Britain, hospital trade unions have emerged from their shadowy existence somewhere in the wings of the National Health Service (NHS) to the center of the political stage. From a situation in which industrial action was virtually unknown, even on wage issues, by 1976 every grade of hospital staff has taken some sort of national strike action, including direct action for and against the retention of private "pay-beds" within NHS hospital wards, strike protest against government welfare policy, pickets of hospital workers against proposed stiffening of the abortion laws, and a multitude of disputes over hours, conditions, and discipline. As inflation and the newfound refusal of NHS employees to subsidize the service by derisory wage levels combine to squeeze the NHS budget, the whole future of our health service is being thrown into question.

The 1945 ideal of a national service, free at the time of use and fully comprehensive, which was in Bevan's words to be "a triumphant example of the superiority of collective action and public initiative applied to a segment of society where commercial principles are seen at their worst" is under challenge. The private health industry, virtually driven out of business with the foundation of a health service where "poverty would not be a disability and wealth not an advantage," is growing once again, newly fortified with multinational capital. A determined element of the medical profession seems bent on reestablishing marketplace medicine over the ruins of the NHS. And in this dilemma, which is nothing less than the future of medicine in Britain, the health trade unions face their greatest challenge and opportunity.

In this brief survey, written in the heat of the first unofficial national industrial action over working hours by junior hospital doctors, I would like to look chronologically at some of the milestones in this new militancy.

The establishment of the NHS brought automatic recognition of the right of all hospital workers to join a union of their choice. The unions, very roughly represented according to membership, meet nationally to negotiate over conditions and service in bodies known as Whitley Councils, ten separate but linked bodies covering the different grades of hospital worker. This method of wage bargaining applies generally in the public sector in Britain and was consciously introduced as a check to the vigorous local bargaining which was the backbone of the syndicalist movement earlier in this century. Although it does guarantee the right to union membership, obviously an advance on the situation in the United States, it tends to put rank-and-file members in an extremely passive position in that they are only nominal members of a union whose annual wage bargaining is conducted in almost incomprehensible complexity by professional management, professional union full-timers, and civil servants.

The main hospital manual unions have tended to reflect this structure. The National Union of Public Employees, with about 90,000 hospital members (including porters, domestic workers, ward cleaners, chefs, cooks, kitchen workers, telephonists, gardeners, laundry workers, and workers in many other manual trades as well as a growing number of nurses), grew out of a union for all London municipal employees founded by a London socialist sewage worker in 1888. By and large, its hospital members simply tagged behind the settlements negotiated with the Local Authority manual workers. Although the Union grew enormously with the foundation of the NHS, the only industrial action it took was in 1956 when mass meetings of women domestics in London forced the Union to take up the struggle for the 44-hour work week which had been granted to every other industry and service in 1953. In most hospitals, Union dues were checked off automatically by management, Union meetings were infrequent, and the officers of the local branch tended to be reelected without change or challenge, often simply because of the status of their hospital job rather than their commitment to unionism. The unelected full-time officers of the Union seemed to see their role as almost philanthropic, looking after "their" hospital workers. The results were exceptionally low basic wages for a fairly demoralized membership who were forced to work enormous lengths of overtime to earn a living wage.

The Confederation of Health Service Employees is in theory the industrial union for the NHS, but in practice its real base is among the predominantly male mental hospital nurses and some of the more senior nurses in the general hospitals. A militant campaigner among the nurses after the establishment of the NHS, the Confederation was recently disaffiliated from the Trades Union Congress during the battle against the Conservative Government's Industrial Relations Act for registering itself on the official government roll which the majority of trade unions were boycotting. The Transport and General Workers Union, the leftish general workers' union, organizes some hospitals, notably in Scotland and the North, but this seems to be a matter of chance. The General and Municipal Workers Union, a notoriously undemocratic and right-wing general union, also has a base in some hospitals. Curiously, these four unions, with widely differing memberships, have equal votes on the Whitley Council covering ancillary workers, which enables the two hospital unions' negotiators to blame the overrepresented general unions for any defect in the annual settlement without actually having to do anything about it themselves.

The nurses, the largest and worst paid category of hospital workers until quite recently, have only rarely joined the industrial unions, preferring instead membership in professional bodies like the Royal College of Nursing and the Royal College of Midwives which combine educational and professional functions with some dabbling in wage negotiation. These bodies are dominated by senior nurses and have no effective and democratic control by student and ward nurses. Hospital clerical workers and administrators also join a mixture of professional and trade union bodies, but the National Association of the Local Government Officers, the militant town hall union, has increasingly become dominant. A scattering of industrial and craft unions cover the skilled manual tradesmen such as electricians, plumbers, builders, and the silver and gold trades workers inside hospitals. These craft unions, which have been increasingly attempting to negotiate wages directly with the Department of Health and Social Security, have often provided a core of trade union experience within the hospitals.

Doctors have traditionally had a different negotiating procedure, the Review Body system. At periodic intervals when professional discontent reaches a certain point, an allegedly independent group of members of the Establishment, usually chaired by a retired managing director, takes evidence from all interested bodies and submits an award to the Prime Minister of the day who can accept, modify, postpone, or reject it.

Despite regular exasperated uprisings and splits, the effectively dominant representative body remains the British Medical Association, not unfairly called the "Tory Party at the bedside." The Junior Hospital Doctors Association emerged in the mid-sixties to dramatize the conditions of house officers doing their compulsory preregistration jobs in a sort of medieval apprenticeship and the long hours, poor residential conditions, and bad educational facilities for registrars (interns) who were still undergoing hospital-based postgraduate specialist education but were more often used as cheap medical labor. More recently the provincial consultants (the heads of the hospital clinical teams) have broken away from what they see as an unrepresentative and London teaching hospital-biased BMA elite. The Medical Practitioners Union, the only genuine trade union operating among doctors, has traditionally been based on the general practitioners, but has recently expanded briskly among more radically minded hospital juniors as part of the general spread of trade unionism among white-collar workers in Britain. The Medical Practitioners Union is now a subsection of the Association of Scientific and Management Staffs, the fastest growing of the white-collar unions which organize in insurance, research, and technical laboratories, but whose membership includes airline pilots, executives, and office workers as well.

Before 1970, despite a fair degree of muttering and grumbling, none of these unions seriously attempted to use industrial action to improve wages or conditions. The emphasis was still on the quality of the negotiators rather than the potential power of the membership. In this respect there was not a great difference between those unions which adopted left-wing resolutions at their annual conferences and those which passed right-wing pronouncements. The bulk of the membership saw union membership as a necessary evil, to give some measure of job security, access to a legal department, and cut-price holidays, domestic appliances, and insurance schemes.

The first sign of a different mood came from the underpaid and underappreciated ancillary workers. In 1970 an unofficial strike broke out in the Royal Free Hospital in London, an establishment founded by women suffragette doctors. The Cinderellas of the hospital service, the porters, theatre technicians, domestics, telephonists, and boilermen, went on a one-day strike, joined by union members in St. Mary's and Bethnal Green Hospitals. The mixture of caution and desperate impatience can be seen in one of the leaflets distributed at the Royal Free Hospital: "We apologize for any inconvenience this may cause you, but as you know our basic wage in the hospital service is scandalous considering today's cost of living, and our conditions of service leave much to be desired, like the fact we have to work seven years before we get three weeks' annual holiday." The basic rates for married hospital workers were still £14, £2.50 under the national minimum wage suggested by the Trades Union Congress.

By the autumn of 1972, many hospital ancillary workers were actually getting basic wages below the official government poverty line and would have done better financially if they had ceased working and drew unemployment and social security benefits. Then all the major hospitals in Bristol were stopped by a walkout, a quite spontaneous revolt which bewildered union full-timers who had hitherto been bemoaning their members' lack of fight. More and more hospitals inspired by the Bristol strikers held special and unusually crowded meetings to discuss action. Union negotiators went back and managed to extract a slightly improved offer, only to find it threatened with inclusion in a 90-day government pay freeze. Hospital workers' natural reluctance to withdraw their labor and concern for patient care was finally overcome with the conviction that the time was ripe to demand attention for the whole plight of the underfinanced health service.

An informal and unofficial rank-and-file body, the London Alliance of Stewards for Health Workers, called for a one-day stoppage on November 27, 1972, and were frankly amazed at the support it received, especially from black women workers who had hitherto largely been excluded from union activity. The strikers demonstrated for hours outside the headquarters of the Department of Health and Social Security in South London chanting, "Hospital pay makes us sick," and hooting the General Secretary of the National Union of Public Employees. The strikers' demands were radical and were determined, if necessary, to break the pay freeze; they called for an all-out strike for an £8 wage increase without strings, a 35-hour week, and 4-week annual paid holidays. Most importantly, the mood was insistent on equal pay for women hospital workers and against productivity deals, i.e. work-measurement bonus schemes which the hospital unions had persistently sold their memberships in lieu of an increase in the basic wage.

The hospital ancillary unions responded by calling an official national one-day strike on December 17, 1972, which had a massive response. An estimated 180,000 went on strike, many for the full 24 hours. In London over 7,000 took part in a demonstration to the Department of Health and Social Security and 500 attended an impromptu meeting held by the London Alliance of Stewards for Health Workers. In the North West of Britain about 200 hospitals came out, with 2,000 marching in Manchester and 1,500 in Liverpool supported by the banners of other trade unions. There was a token sit-in at the Department of Health and Social Security Regional Office by 150 people while a deputation took in a protest letter.

The catering staff in Oldham cut back on private patients' luxurious meals for the duration of the action. Ancillary staff in the North East were obstructed by management in their efforts to organize an emergency service and as a result pulled out completely in nine hospitals. Five hundred marched in Newcastle, 3,000 in the Midlands, 1,500 in Sheffield, a total of 5,000 in Wales, and 2,000 in Bristol. In Scotland 7,000 workers from 48 Glasgow hospitals were joined on their march by striking domestic staff members from Stirling University. On the strength of this feeling, the unions began official ballotting over strike action and the London Alliance of Stewards for Health Workers extended itself, for a brief period, to a national rank-and-file organization and published a paper called "Backlash."

By February 1973, after an exceptionally complex and long-winded ballotting procedure and another burst of unofficial action again led by transport union members in Bristol (who this time stayed out for four days before officials persuaded them to go back with promises of official action), national action was announced. But in contrast with the ballot's emphatic call for an all-out strike by over half the members, the unions called for a series of half measures: selective strikes, to be coordinated from the head office, an overtime ban, and "withdrawal of cooperation." The strategy, if it existed, was to allow strong branches to take the brunt of the attack while allowing the less militant areas to choose their own tactics according to their confidence. And in the first two weeks of March, British hospitals were shaken to their foundations. The first national strike surprised everyone, the Tories, the hospital administrators, the consultants, and many hospital workers themselves, with its determination and spirit. The picket-line posters put it plainly with the slogans "We are against the government not the patients" and "Hospital workers stick together."

Women workers, scarcely represented in the union hierarchy and always blamed by male union officials as the reason there was never any militant action, led many of the strikes and marches. At one Birmingham hospital, women pickets succeeded in turning away lorry drivers at one gate who promptly drove down the road and talked their way in through the male picket line. Workers of all languages, colors, and nationalities were joined together, and signs in picket lines were in Italian, Greek, Spanish, and even Gaelic. Over 400 hospitals had strikes ranging from one-day strikes to all-out stoppages. A cluster of sit-ins took place in response to management attempts to bring in volunteers. Selective action in laundries and sterilizing depots began to put direct pressure on the ability of many hospitals to keep even an emergency service open, and nine hospital boards wrote to Sir Keith Joseph, the responsible Minister, asking him to pay the wage increases at once.

But as the strike dragged on, although morale stayed high where effective action was taken, financial pressure built up on the hospital workers' very small cash resources, and the mosaic-like pattern of action became confusing and demoralizing. Solidarity action was hard to organize. In some cases the hospital workers had already been forced back to work by the time their industrial supporters were ready to take sympathy action. The rank-and-file organizations were engulfed, and strikers had to rely on the papers or their union full-timers, both with their own biases, or set up their own coordination centers, sometimes based on strike bulletins like "Flying Picket," the Camden Public Sector Alliance "Bulletin," or the Leeds "Hospital Worker."

Enthusiasm was replaced by frustration and tears, and when the Tories and the unions arrived at a face-saving formula, most strikers were glad to return to work. For although the cash reward was pathetic, more important points had been made—that hospital workers were no longer going to allow their dedication to be exploited and that the miracles of medicine performed by the consultants in their white coats were only possible because of a whole series of invisible, unglamorous, but absolutely essential supporting workers. Without packers in the hospital sterilization units, people to burn the rubbish, and ladies to pour the tea, even the most prestigious hospital ground to a halt. Many of the consultants who had denounced the strike action from the comfort of their limousines were to regret their remarks.

And even out of the technical defeat of the strike, a new mood of determination surfaced in the branches. For every member who disgustedly tore up his union card, there were ten who rolled up their sleeves and decided to build an organization that would be ready for the next round. Union membership swelled, especially the National Union of Public Employees, and a new national rank-and-file paper, "Hospitalworker," was founded by a delegate conference in Birmingham and sponsored by over 40 leading rank and filers. The mood had altered for good; within weeks the Nurses Action Group was leafleting nurses' homes with the message, "Professionalism means nothing when we are used as cheap labor. We are doing a hard skilled job and we do it because we care. We also care when we are unable to do it properly because of lack of manpower and inevitable falling standards in a crumbling Health Service." In autumn of 1973, ambulancemen followed the defiant Scottish firemen in challenging phase 3 of the Tory pay code, and using their traditions of militancy and high mobility they achieved a substantial increase. "What is it worth to pick up the dead?" one poster asked starkly.

One of the tactics discovered in the 1973 ancillary strike, the selective pressure on the private patients who use NHS facilities while being nursed in separate wings of the public hospitals, was to take on new significance. These NHS pay-beds, only allowed because of a compromise at the foundation of the NHS, were to become a central issue in the two 1974 elections. Hospital unionists argued that their continued existence and the privileges they represented, notably queue-jumping, represented a blatant defiance of the whole idea of equal access to health, while many consultants saw the beds as a legitimate exercise of clinical freedom and a welcome boost to hospital finances. National Union of Public Employees members in Portsmouth and the industrial North West, acting on what had become official union policy since 1973, introduced a ban on pay-beds; a similar ban became front-page news when workers in the new Charing Cross Hospital in London took it up in July 1974.

The British Medical Association took up the challenge and announced a national "work to rule" by hospital consultants; there was much talk of consultants leaving the NHS, setting up their own private medical service, or emigrating from Britain to practice abroad. *The Times* reported that "Industry and big business are interested in providing money to keep the private patients' service going because of the convenience of having their employees looked at and treated quickly."

In the meantime medical technicians in the Association of Scientific and Management Staffs struck and were shortly joined by hospital radiographers. By July 1974

NHS engineering workers joined the cascade. The official doctors' organizations were still adamant over private practice and the general practitioners began a campaign to refuse prescriptions for contraceptives and demote some of their registered list of NHS patients, say all those whose surnames begin with a designated letter, to the status of temporary patients. The letter pages of general practitioners' periodicals were buzzing with ingenious schemes to put pressure on government by refusing the numerous administrative responsibilities required of general practitioners. By the summer months most sections of the NHS had taken action, including 50,000 doctors, 11,000 dentists, 370,000 nurses (who succeeded in Wales and Manchester in bringing out miners and engineers in sympathy strikes under the slogan "Strike a blow for the nurses"), 4,700 radiographers, 4,500 physiotherapists, 1,600 occupational therapists, 350 dietitians, 200 speech therapists, 250 remedial gymnasts, 270 orthopedists, and 150 chiropodists. It was a strike wave which would have seemed impossible only four years earlier, and for a period it was impossible to open a newspaper without seeing a striking hospital worker in uniform striding across it. The Halsbury Report, which was produced to settle the majority of the technical and paramedical staff's claims, was forced to award sizable settlements although they were highly stratified and, in fact, gave comparatively little to the junior grades. It was from this summer of hospital discontent that the Minister made her promise to the hospital junior doctors of a 40-hour basic work week. The complete failure to achieve any real shortening of hours and the refusal to make available new overtime payments to carry out this pledge, justified by reference to national "anti-inflation" policy, are the causes of the strike action being taken in 1975 by the junior doctors. And at the senior end of the medical hierarchy, the consultants have initiated "emergency-only" restrictions in an attempt to block the separation of private and NHS medicine by the phased government removal of hospital pay-beds. This action has in turn stimulated renewed selective action *against* the pay-beds by manual unions. The local government union has begun a campaign to block planning permission to the mushrooming new private hospitals now on the drawing board, if necessary by campaigning in the construction unions for the "blocking" of private hospital building.

Such a sketchy and partial survey can only give the surface impression of what has been an exciting five years. What is clear is that the days of passive, somnambulent dues collecting are bypassed for good by what is a highly political and vigorous trade unionism. On the national scale, strike action has made politics of health care the subject of daily discussion. It is to be hoped that in the next five years British hospital trade unionists will actually come up with some new solutions to problems which for too long have been obscured by the "medical mystique."

PART 2

Allied Workers,
Nurses, Women

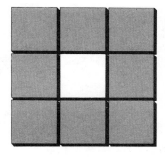

CHAPTER 9

The Division Of Laborers:
Allied Health Professions

Carol A. Brown

The health industry is historically peculiar in the extent to which increased capitalization and mass production led to an increase in craft organization, i.e. a multitude of specialized occupations, whose control and direction rest outside the employing organization, and in which the relations between workers of different occupations (the integration of labor) are governed as much by power relations among professional societies as by organizational managers. The health industry contains over 20 recognized corporate[1] occupations, including medicine with 20 incorporated specialties (2).

Unlike traditional craft industries (such as construction) whose unions are independent of one another, the crafts and professions of health services are hierarchically ordered and controlled. Physicians as a corporate group have power over the allied health professions, e.g. radiologic and medical technology and physical and occupational therapy. The hierarchies of occupations headed by nursing and dentistry are simpler but similar in forms of control. The top occupation acts through a variety of industry-wide organizations to maintain a division of labor to its advantage. In medicine, such bodies include the American Medical Association (AMA), the American Hospital Association (AHA), the Joint Commission on Accreditation of Hospitals (JCAH), the Council on Medical Education (CME), and the American Association of Medical Colleges (AAMC). We will concentrate in this paper on the medical hierarchy, with examples from radiologic technology and medical (clinical laboratory) technology (3).

How the division of labor evolves has been little studied by American sociologists (see Vollmer and Mills (4), Etzioni (5), and Moore (6)). Where attention has been paid,

The material in this paper was prepared under a grant from the Manpower Administration, U.S. Department of Labor, under the authority of Title I of the Manpower Development and Training Act of 1962. Researchers undertaking such projects under government sponsorship are encouraged to express freely their professional judgment. Therefore, points of view or opinions stated in this document do not necessarily represent the official position or policy of the Department of Labor.

[1] The use of the term "corporate" follows Weber's definition (1) of a formally organized body. Occupations having unions, guilds, and professional societies exemplify corporate occupations.

sociologists tend to assume a voluntaristic consensus model, in which people decide to specialize for the sake of efficiency or market expansion. This model is based on the writings of Durkheim (7), and was previously described by Marx (8) as "a posteriori" division, and by Weber (1) as "natural" division. Useful analyses in the health field include Bucher and Strauss (9), Freidson (10), and Moore (6). With great enough differentiation the specialties come to be socially recognized as separate occupations. Under certain circumstances the members of the occupation will decide to raise their status by professionalizing (11, 12).

A more useful model recognizes the importance of power, conflict, and exploitation (1, 8). The model that Marx (8) called "a priori" and Weber "rational" assumes that the division of labor can be controlled, planned, and imposed on the working population by those with organized economic power, and that this model characterizes capitalist industrial society. Marx points out that the division of labor will be shaped to the benefit of the powerful, and that the working population will in turn organize itself in its own interest. Applying this model to the relations among professions in the health services helps to explain many developments.

THE DEVELOPMENT OF LABOR

We first have to consider why health services were conducive to an occupationally dominated division of labor. Health services have been and still are basically a labor-intensive skill industry with workers dispersed in relatively small organizations. The means of production are the applied skills, knowledge, and labor of people rather than of machines. Therefore, efforts to create, change, monopolize, or benefit from a relation to the means of production require direct and conscious intervention in the occupational structure (13, 14). Although control over capital is important, it is not sufficient to control the market.

The historically successful efforts of physicians, as a corporate group, to monopolize the market through governmental imposition of licensing laws are well known (10, 15). We need only point out that monopoly could not be accomplished by permitting a free market.

The 20th century has seen an enormous expansion of the market through technologic developments, the infusion of capital concentrated in hospitals, and expansion of financial support of services. Expansion of the industry has meant an enormous increase in the need for labor with a variety of technical skills (16-18). Although physicians remain the only occupational group which can legally practice medicine, the expansion has taken place not through an increase in number of physicians to cover the increased work (thereby diluting the returns from the market), but by the controlled development of lower status, more narrowly specialized, and much lower paid occupations on a mass basis. While radiologists and pathologists average around $25,000 a year, medical technologists earn about $8,500, and radiologic technologists, $7,000.

That the specialized occupations are controlled by superior occupations, and that the occupations compete with each other are both due to the profit-based economic system, in which one's benefit depends on another's loss. Despite the constantly rising expenditures on health services, consumer spending is not illimitable. Physicians therefore have an incentive not to do the work themselves[2] but to have it done for them by others at lower wages. However, many subordinate health occupations are potentially low-wage substitutes for physicians. Each set of technologists and technicians working under a medical specialist is more highly skilled within the specialty than are physicians who do not specialize in that area. To assure that the subordinate occupations remain subordinates for the superiors' benefit, and not competitors to the superiors' disadvantage, physicians as a corporate group have attempted to keep the subordinates under control, to protect the privileged position of the profession of medicine as a whole.

Although it appears that physicians are losing relative power because of the growth of hospitals and the transfer of market control to larger organizations, the actions of the physicians themselves would argue otherwise. As physicians lost direct control over production organizations, they gained control over the producers, through the AHA, JCAH, CME, and Medicare regulations. Hospital-based physicians have reacted more favorably than physicians in private practice to the development and professionalization of subordinate occupations. In part, this is because hospital physicians feel that their hierarchical position is well protected by industrial regulations, and in part because the costs of improved production do not come directly out of the hospital physicians' pockets.

The subordinate occupations have not functioned entirely for the benefit of physicians. Workers involved in similar employment who share a relation to the means of production will inevitably organize on their own behalf. In Marxian terms, hospital workers have partly become proletarianized, but they have also become "bourgeoisified," by accepting the physicians' model of professional incorporation, licensure, educational control, and employment monopoly, and by competing for the same occupational space. Each subordinate occupation has an incentive to divide itself from other occupations and defend its territory from encroachment. In addition, the government, the educational system, and the market (in terms of patients and third parties) have their own ideas about how the labor and the benefits from labor should be divided. This obviously leads to an extremely complex set of conflicts over occupations.

A description of the occupational interrelations is in order. Since a complete description would be beyond the scope of this paper, we will try to give a general overview with examples.

PROFESSIONAL SOCIETIES

The AMA acts somewhat as a holding company for the corporate profession of medicine, with each specialty having its own college and perhaps a subspecialty association. Each allied health profession has its own professional society, most of which were developed by the medical profession and are formally linked to the AMA or the specialty college. For example, the American Society of Radiologic

---

[2] Physicians have based their claims to privilege on their greater skill and training which protect the patient. Were this indeed the argument, either they would not be willing to entrust patients to less trained personnel, or they would recognize the greater skills of subordinates by giving them higher positions.

Technologists (ASRT) was founded in 1920 after negotiation with radiologists (19). The registry of trained professionals was begun in 1922 under the auspices of ASTR, the American College of Radiology (ACR), the American Roentengen Ray Society (which quickly withdrew), and the Radiological Society of America which withdrew in favor of ACR shortly before World War II (20). By 1951, requirements for becoming a registered x-ray technician had changed from proof of employment in an x-ray organization to proof of a year's training under a radiologist. By 1966, graduation from a 2-year school certified by ACR, in a hospital accredited by JCAH, became the only entry route. Thus the radiology profession gained ever greater control over radiologic technology as the subordinate profession developed.

In both radiology and pathology, the specialists have a measure of direct and indirect authority over the internal machinery of their respective technologists. The commissions on technician affairs of the specialty organizations review decisions by the technologist societies. The specialist societies provide an important portion of the finances for the technologist societies. In addition, the elected officers of the technologist societies are employed by individual specialists, who must provide some expenses and some time off to these employees.

Charters of the technologist societies allow them to be concerned only with educational matters. Technologists must subscribe to highly restrictive codes of ethics required by ACR, the College of American Pathology (CAP), and the AMA. Thus, technologists may work only for members of the medical profession; they may teach technology only in an accredited training school directed by a specialist; they may not own or work in a private laboratory. Failure to comply with the code results in loss of professional registration.

EDUCATION AND TRAINING

Control over the education and training of a profession's members means control over the production of workers and thus over the division of labor. Educational power includes determining the content and duration of training, monopolizing the auspices under which training takes place, selecting the trainees, and certifying the graduates.

The AMA Council on Medical Education is empowered by the United States Office of Education, via the National Accrediting Commission, to approve curricula, accredit schools, and certify graduates in the medical profession and in eight subordinate professions. Training usually must take place in an accredited hospital in a CME-approved school. The CME can slow, if not halt, an occupation's development by refusing to accredit its training programs, and has used its legal power to prevent the development of alternative training and accrediting systems. For example, the CME blocked private trade schools from accrediting medical office assistants.

Even health occupations that are not directly controlled by CME are subject to limitation by the medical profession. The JCAH can and has threatened to withdraw its accreditation from hospitals which offer training in unacceptable occupations. The AAMC and individual medical colleges control acess to the necessary clinical training facilities in teaching hospitals and university medical centers, and can agree or refuse to allow training for developing occupations. The development of nurse-midwifery has been slowed by the reluctance of hospitals and medical schools to approve training programs. Obstetricians have been most active in blocking the development of this occupation.

Medical schools have actively developed new occupations such as the recent "physician assistants," who appear to be the medical profession's answer to the nurses' "clinical specialists." The spread of a new occupation depends largely on its acceptance by the most important medical school complexes. Among the occupations recently created and trained in medical centers are inhalation therapists, electroencephalograph technicians, orthoptists, orthotists and prosthetists, mental health technicians, physical therapy technicians, medical records technicians, and cytotechnologists.

Boards of registry approve training and certify graduates in each occupation. Registries of subordinate professions are not necessarily controlled by their own members. The medical technologist registry has been a standing committee of the American Society of Clinical Pathologists (ASCP). Even when nominally independent of superiors, the actions of the registries are subject to approval by CME and the House of Delegates of the AMA, which will both heed the advice of the relevant medical specialty. Curricula of the schools are carefully controlled to produce those skills needed in subordinates but not those which might compete with superiors.

The kinds of conflicts that take place over education and the reasons for them can be seen in the clinical laboratory field. Officially recognized as subordinate to the clinical pathologists is the profession of medical technologists, MT(ASCP). At a time when 84 per cent of registered MTs had 3 or more years of college prior to clinical training, the official ASCP prerequisite was only 2 years of college, thus essentially defining away wage claims that might be made on the grounds of education (21). Through lobbying by the American Society of Medical Technologists (ASMT) with ASCP and CAP, the requirements were raised to 3 and finally, to 4 years.

Technicians, workers with some college education, were never officially recognized, nor were laboratory assistants who had no formal education. ASMT developed the Certified Laboratory Assistant and Histologic Technologist programs requiring 1 year of training under a medical technologist, which qualified high school graduates to perform simple laboratory jobs under direction of a technologist. These programs would have the effect of eliminating technician competition and creating an unbridgeable gap between responsible MTs and all lower level workers.

ASCP was unenthusiastic about these programs. As conflict between ASCP and the American Society of Medical Technologists (ASMT) grew over this and other issues, pathologists came to desire a less competitive and less costly but still skilled set of subordinates. ASCP directed its Boards of Schools and of Registry to work out accredited junior college programs for technicians under the auspices of ASCP. ASCP would, in effect, be creating a subordinate occupation that would undercut its recognized subordinates.

ASMT countered by demanding independence of the Boards from ASCP. Neither an industrial mediator nor a study committee of AMA was able to settle the issues. ASMT began outflanking the pathologists by opening membership to unregistered college graduate technologists and scientists, and by signing "treaties of friendship" with previously disdained technician associations. ASCP moved to reassert control over the Boards, and began withdrawing its financial support from ASMT and the National

Committee for Careers in Medical Technology. ASMT considered suing ASCP and CAP as combinations in restraint of trade.

INDUSTRIAL RULES AND REGULATIONS

Much occupational control takes place through what might be called the industrial rules and regulations, the private government of an industry whose actions have quasi-legal power. The medical profession, through its private regulatory power over hospitals, not only commands the major capital concentrations in the health services industry but also has a measure of control over other occupations which are dependent on hospital employment.

The division of labor within hospitals is not regulated by the local hospital administrator or medical board, but nationally by JCAH. JCAH is a joint body of AMA, AHA, and the American College of Surgeons, all exclusively or partially composed of physicians.[3] The power of JCAH to accredit hospitals is legally sanctioned by the U.S. Public Health Service which dispenses construction and reimbursement funds, and by state and local health agencies which control operating licenses. Accrediting standards include a staffing guide regulating what positions may be held by members of what occupations. A board-certified medical specialist must control each medical service, and "appropriate" numbers of allied health profession members must be hired. Various occupations are forbidden entry. For many years clinical scientists (Ph.D. chemists, microbiologists, etc.) were kept out of the direction of hospital laboratories by JCAH.[4]

The staffing regulations do not work entirely in favor of the recognized subordinate professions. Only "appropriate" numbers of them need to be hired, mandating in effect an open shop for labor. Thus the professional status of the lower occupations is dependent in part on the willingness of employers to recognize and hire them. Physicians set the employment qualifications within the medical services as well as in their private practices. Since large numbers of non-professionals are in fact hired, it becomes apparent that the medical profession is not that willing to pay for the highly skilled manpower whose development it officially supports.

Other professional associations publish hospital staffing guidelines, but lack power to impose them. The development of licensed practical nursing training, and the mass employment of licensed practical nurses and nurses aides over the opposition of registered nurses, is a case in point. Assistant occupations in physical and occupational therapy have been developed in medical centers with government manpower training funds over the objections of therapist professional societies.

LICENSING

The practice of medicine laws have been used to block the development of organizations and occupations not under control of physicians. Within the past year

[3] The absence of the American Nursing Association, representing the key occupations in hospital work, is noteworthy.

[4] Because of this, many clinical scientists went into public health service. With the increased importance of government funding, clinical scientists are often in a position to regulate their erstwhile regulators.

these laws have been used to close a women's self-help clinic in Los Angeles and an acupuncture clinic in New York City. Radiologists used medical practice acts to abolish private x-ray laboratories, and pathologists' inability to do the same with private clinical laboratories has led to continuing conflict.[5] CAP has been sued by the U.S. Department of Justice as a combination in restraint of trade for its efforts to eliminate private competition.

By controlling the employing organizations, the medical profession controls the occupations whose members might work there. A monopsony, or monopoly over employment opportunities, enables employers to control an occupation and to force salaries downward. Hospital collusion to keep wage rates down has been found in nursing (22). One of the more highly paid professions in health is medical social work, which is peripheral to strictly medical functions but offers the greatest alternative employment opportunities (23.) Members of both of the technology professions which we examined are by AMA regulations forbidden to work under the auspices of non-physicians or to become self-employed. Medical technologists have broken this regulation through a costly court battle over registration privileges. A survey by ASMT (21) showed that median MT salaries in industry and independent laboratories were almost a thousand dollars higher than in hospitals. Radiologic technologists have nowhere else to go.

Other forms of governmental control have been used by the medical profession (24). Guidelines for Medicare reimbursements were written to give automatic acceptance to JCAH standards, and to favor various medical specialties. At one time reimbursements for mental health treatment by clinical psychologists were denied unless that treatment had been prescribed by a physician. Staffing regulations were written for private laboratories receiving Medicare funds; however, pathologists gained across-the-board exemptions for their own laboratories, whether in or out of hospitals, and required that the top staff for private laboratories be trained in pathologist-directed laboratories (25).

Occupational licensing is a more direct means of control over an occupation (26, 27). Since a license legally establishes a division of labor, it is in the interest of an occupation to gain licensure for itself and to have its professional requirements serve as the basis for licensure. It is also in an occupation's interest to prevent the licensure of its competitors or subordinates. As long as professional registration of subordinates remains under AMA auspices, physicians can choose to accept or reject the professionally trained and higher cost subordinates, and can alter the training system to suit themselves. Licensing of subordinates cuts out the alternative of hiring cheap workers and carries the risk of losing control over the subordinate occupation to the subordinates themselves or to the state.

Physicians have campaigned repeatedly and often sucessfully to prevent the licensure of lower level professions. Failing that, physicians have attempted to control the licensure of their employees. Many subordinate health occupations have physicians on their licensing boards, often as majorities (28). Often AMA-approved certification is considered sufficient qualification for licensing.

The state medical practice acts take priority over other health licenses. The

---

[5] Performing the routine x-ray procedures does not require a physician any more than does the performance of a laboratory test. Technologists are usually more capable of accurate test performance than are most physicians. Interpreting the results is the medical procedure which must be performed by a physician in both the laboratory and x-ray fields.

subordinates' license prevents anyone *but a physician* from performing the subordinates' work. The physician need not have training in the specialized area. The medical practice acts have also been interpreted to permit physician control over the work of other subordinate occupations. Technicians, nurses, and others may perform "medical" tasks, but their right to perform the tasks and to hold jobs in which such tasks are performed usually rests with the state medical practice board (28). The subordinate is usually limited to working under the financial control or direction of physicians.

Licensing changes the division of labor: who "wins" and who "loses" is not always clear, as shown in examples from radiologic and medical technology.

The first licensing law for radiologic technologists, in New York State, was opposed by both ACR and ASRT, who rightly feared loss of control over technologists. The state system is modelled on the ACR system (thus preventing charges of "dilution of quality") with the minute difference that it is mandatory, not voluntary, and under state control. Among the immediate effects of the law were the following: several ACR-approved schools were closed due to "poor quality" (29); state-approved schools directed by licensed technologists were opened in community colleges, not under ACR auspices[6]; a few registered technologists were refused licenses on grounds of incompetence; over 6000 persons who had previously taken x-rays (nurses aides, physician's office assistants, part-time and untrained technicians) were eliminated from that area of work and had to be replaced by licensed technologists. Hospitals and radiologists in private practice benefitted from the increased business sent to them by private practitioners who could not afford to hire the trained and licensed technologists. The state also mandated staffing regulations for hospital radiology departments, thus opening higher level administrative positions to technologists than had previously been available.

Despite continuing objections by ACR and ASRT, technologists in other states began licensure campaigns. ACR countered by suggesting a federal license based solely on the Registry. ACR convinced several state technologist societies to drop their state licensure drives and, instead, to push for federal licensure. ACR then dropped its federal licensure drive. Several states now have mandatory licensure for radiologic technologists.

A slightly different licensure effort affected clinical laboratories in New York City, to the detriment of almost every profession. The New York City Bureau of Laboratories, staffed largely by clinical scientists and headed by an M.D. with a Ph.D., imposed regulations that did not accept any profession's model, but created instead five levels of workers according to five levels of education, from high school graduate to doctoral degree. By giving equal weight to medical-professional training and to non-medical academic training, they removed the former privileges enjoyed by all the professions under the medical system. By requiring that all laboratories have working directors and full-time supervision, and that no person work above the level of his license, the Bureau's regulations effectively blocked previously available opportunities for technicians and technologists to rise into administration or self-employment, and created a stratification system based on access to higher education.

Pathologists, like the radiologists, have considered moving their level of governmental control upward. They managed to prevent adoption of the New York

---

[6] ACR subsequently ruled their graduates ineligible for professional certification.

City model under Medicare and secured a federal act requiring federal licensure of all hospital and independent laboratories (2). Accreditation by CAP's Commission on Laboratory Inspection and Accreditation, composed of its own members, was made sufficient for licensure. Since hospital laboratories are already under JCAH and CAP control, and pathologist-directed laboratories in private practice are exempt from the licensure, the pathologists will, in essence, have licensing control over their competitors.

CONCLUSION

We have seen the various ways in which the medical profession asserts control over subordinate occupations, as well as efforts by the subordinate occupations on their own behalf. What does this auger for the future?

There is an increasing tendency to believe that physicians are losing control of health services, as hospitals and financial organizations come into dominance. It is my belief that physicians are not the endangered species some think they are. The general practitioner is definitely on his way out, and the ability of the AMA to protect private practice is in decline. But, as the medical profession changes, its organizations of control also change. The combined power of the AMA, JCAH, CME, AAMC, and AHA is very strong. The chances of any other occupation taking over control of the health industry and becoming the top ranking profession are slim.

Physicians retain control over industrial production, in large part because of their control over other workers. The more hospital-centered health services become, the greater will be the elaboration of occupations over which physicians have hegemony, and the greater the elaboration of control machinery.

Subordinate occupations are fighting for more space, but this does not argue a revolt of the proletariat. If anything, it argues a successful "bourgeoisification" of labor along medical lines, and a bulwark against unionism.[7] It also represents a "triumph of conservatism" (30), since, as physicians lose direct control, they gain regulatory power.

Such a system is neither efficient nor favorable to the public interest. Medicine for profit leads inevitably to conflict over occupational territories, to distortion of the division of labor for the sake of income rather than service, and results in either the exploitation of workers through low wages or the exploitation of consumers through high prices. Far preferable would be a socialist division of labor among occupations and organizations whose cooperative interaction would serve everyone's needs.

REFERENCES

1. Weber, M. *Theory of Social and Economic Organization,* edited by T. Parsons, pp. 2-54. Free Press of Glencoe, London, 1964.

[7] The chairman of the Committee on Technician Affairs of the American College of Radiology said: "Much of the agitation for licensing of x-ray technicians and for unionization stems from the abuses and exploitation of students in training schools and from technologists who resent the lack of interest of radiologists in their educational and financial welfare. Better trained and better paid technologists have a more professional attitude and are less likely to seek unionization and licensing as solutions for their problems. They also more properly appreciate their role in medicine and their relationship to their radiologists" (20).

2. United States Public Health Service. *Health Resources Statistics, Health Manpower and Health Facilities 1970*, Publication No. 1509, 1970.
3. Brown, C.A. Development of Occupations in Health Technology. Unpublished dissertation, Columbia University, 1971.
4. Vollmer, H., and Mills, D., editor. *Professionalization*. Prentice-Hall, Inc., Englewood Cliffs, New Jersey, 1966.
5. Etzioni, A., editor. *The Semi-Professions and Their Organization*. Free Press, New York, 1969.
6. Moore, W. *The Professions: Roles and Rules*. Russell Sage Foundation, New York, 1970.
7. Durkheim, E. *The Division of Labor in Society*. Free Press of Glencoe, London, 1964.
8. Marx, K. *Capital*, pp. 368-394. Modern Library, New York, 1960.
9. Bucher, R., and Strauss, A. Professions in process. *Am. J. Sociol.* 66:325-334, 1961.
10. Freidson, E. *Professional Dominance*. Atherton Press, New York, 1970.
11. Goode, W.J. The Theoretical Limits of Professionalization. In *The Semi-Professions and Their Organization*, edited by A. Etzioni. Free Press, New York, 1969.
12. Wilensky, H. The professionalization of everyone? *Am. J. Sociol.* 70: 137-158, 1964.
13. Kerr, C. The Balkanization of Labor Markets. In *Labor Mobility and ,Economic Opportunity*, edited by E. Bakke, P. Hauser, et al. Technology Press of MIT and John Wiley & Sons, Inc., New York, 1954.
14. Kerr, C., and Siegal, A. The structuring of the labor force in industrial society: New dimensions and new questions. *Industrial and Labor Relations Review* 8: 151-168, 1955.
15. Rayack, E. *Professional Power and American Medicine*. World Publishing Company, New York, 1967.
16. Greenfield, H.I., and Brown, C.A. *Allied Health Manpower: Trends and Prospects*. Columbia University Press, New York, 1969.
17. Sturm, H. M. Technological developments and their effect upon health manpower. *Monthly Labor Review* 90, 1967.
18. Somers, H., and Somers, A. *Doctors, Patients and Health Insurance*. Anchor Books, Garden City, 1962.
19. Greene, A. B. Quo fata vocant? *X-Ray Technician* 26: 76-88, 1954.
20. Soule, A. B. Trends in training programs in radiologic technology. *Radiol. Technol.* 38: 70-73, 1966.
21. Salaries Continue to Rise. *GIST*, A Newsletter relating to the Profession of Medical Technology, No. 36, April 1967.
22. Klarman, H. *Hospital Care in New York City*. Columbia University Press, New York, 1963.
23. United States Department of Labor. *Hospitals, March 1969*. Industry Wage Survey, Bulletin 1688, 1969.
24. Gilb, C. L. *Hidden Hierarchies: The Professions and Government*. Harper and Row, New York, 1966.
25. United States Social Security Administration. *Conditions for Coverage of Independent Laboratories*. HIR 13, 1968.
26. Rottenberg, S. The Economics of Occupational Licensing. In *Aspects of Labor Economics*. National Bureau of Economic Research, Special Conference Series No. 14. Princeton University Press, Princeton, 1962.
27. Friedman, M. *Capitalism and Freedom*. University of Chicago Press, Chicago, 1962.
28. United States Public Health Service. *State Licensing of Health Occupations*. Publication No. 1758, 1967.
29. Goldman, H. Licensure of X-Ray Technicians in New York State. New York State Department of Health, 1968 (mimeograph).
30. Kolko, G. *The Triumph of Conservatism*. Free Press of Glencoe, London, 1963.

CHAPTER 10

The Development Of The Nursing Labor Force In The United States: A Basic Analysis

Kathleen Cannings and William Lazonick

The United States health system is controlled by and run in the interests of an elite consisting of hospital and nursing home employers, an upper stratum of the medical profession, and the large corporate capitalists of the pharmaceutical, insurance, and medical supplies industries. Although this elite of health employers has reciprocated with the delivery of a mass of products in the form of health care service and medications, their monopolistic control of the various parts of the health industry has clearly become detrimental to the quality and quantity of health care available to the people of the U.S. (1-4). In this paper, we will not dwell on the nature of the output of the health industry, but rather on the characteristics of the work relations within the industry which make the output possible. In particular, we will focus on the development of the nursing labor force in a health system over which nursing workers have hitherto had virtually no control.

In 1972, the employed nursing labor force in the U.S. was composed of 780,000 registered nurses, 427,000 practical nurses, and about 900,000 nursing aides, orderlies, attendants, and home health aides. They constituted about 48 per cent of the approximately 4.4 million people employed in the U.S. health industry and about 68 per cent of the health workers rendering direct aid to patients (5, pp. 8-11). It is from the surplus labor of these nursing workers that the financial gains of employers in the health care industry are increasingly derived. These employers, on the one hand, utilize the services of these wage-workers (i.e. workers who are paid by doctors and hospitals rather than by the actual consumers of health care), and, on the other hand, pocket the health care fees paid by the consumers. Although the high incomes of doctors are to some extent due to the restriction of their own labor supply, the major source of the high profits and incomes of the elite of the health industry lies in the labor of the nursing labor force.

As we shall see, the nursing labor force, under the control of this elite, has taken on an increasing role (both in terms of absolute labor-time and relative to doctors) in the *actual delivery* of health care. Without these workers, the health employers would not be able to market the mass of health services from which they make their financial gains and by which they maintain their power. In this social relation lie both the present weakness and the potential strength of the nursing labor force in shaping both their own lives and the delivery of health care. Historically, the health employers have gained increasing control over the working lives of the nursing labor force and over the character of the health services which that labor force provides and which it is able to provide. But, at the same time, in the process of achieving that control, the power of health employers has become more and more dependent on their ability to reproduce that control in the workplaces (and schools) of the health industry.

The nursing labor force, because it occupies such a key position in the actual delivery of health care, is in a *potentially* powerful position to keep health employers from reproducing that control. As in other work processes in capitalist society, the subjugation of the mass of laborers in the interests of the private gain of those few who control the means of labor is, in essence, the denial of the right of workers to control the use of their own labor and the product of their labor. This "right" will only come to those workers who collectively develop sufficient political power to take control of their own work processes.

In this paper, we do not attempt, except in the most general way, to analyze how the nursing labor force might develop that power. Rather, we draw together some basic material on the objective character of the nursing labor force which may be helpful in beginning that analysis. In the first section of the paper, we present a statistical and descriptive picture of the nursing labor force as it exists today. In the second section, we sketch the historical development of that labor force up to about 1950, stressing its general integration into a hierarchical and concentrated health industry. In the third and final section, we present a more detailed analysis of the quantitative and qualitative development of the nursing labor force over the past 25 years.

THE NURSING LABOR FORCE

Worker Characteristics

There are three outstanding characteristics of the nursing labor force as it exists in the 1970s. It is composed predominantly of women, it is highly stratified, and most work is performed in large institutional settings. There are three broad categories of nursing workers: registered nurses (RNs), practical (or vocational) nurses (PNs), and nursing aides (including orderlies and attendants) (NAs). In 1972, there were approximately 780,000 employed registered nurses in the U.S., 98.6 per cent of whom were women; about 427,000 employed practical nurses, 97 per cent of whom were women; and about 900,000 employed nursing aides, orderlies, attendants, and home health aides, 80-85 per cent of whom were women. Table 1 shows the distribution of these workers among the various types of workplaces (6).

These three categories of the nursing labor force shade into one another in terms of the type of work performed, while within the RN group itself there is a highly stratified and hierarchical division of labor. It is mainly through educational credentials and licensure (or lack of it) that workers are channelled into these three categories.

Table 1

Percentage distribution of the nursing labor force in the U.S., by place of work, 1972[a]

Workers	Hospitals	Nursing Homes	Public Health	Other[b]	Total
RNs	65.2	7.0	9.0	18.8	100.0
PNs	63.2	17.1	0.9	18.7	100.0
NAs[c]	66.3	31.1	2.3	0.2	100.0
All nursing workers	65.3	19.4	4.5	10.8	100.0

[a]Source, reference 6, Tables I-A-6, IV-A-1, IV-B-1.
[b]Includes occupational health, nursing education, private duty, office.
[c]Nursing aides, orderlies, attendants, and home health aides.

There are no definite educational requirements for NAs, but almost all undergo on-the-job training programs usually of four to six weeks in duration. Practical nurses usually have 12 months of training which is received primarily in vocational schools and junior colleges. Most PNs are licensed by a state licensing board. Registered nurses, who are also licensed by their own state boards, must complete two years of postsecondary schooling to receive an associate degree (A.D.) from a community college or three years for a diploma from a hospital-based nursing school. A growing proportion of RNs are completing B.S. degrees in nursing at four-year colleges, and some of these graduates are going on to master's and doctoral programs in nursing. In 1971–1972, out of a total of 51,784 graduates from initial registered nursing programs, 41.7 per cent graduated from hospital-based diploma courses, 37.0 per cent graduated from community college-based associate degree courses, and 21.3 per cent graduated from college and university-based baccalaureate programs in nursing (6, Table II-A-6). In addition, in 1971–1972, 4,499 RNs who had already graduated from one of these initial programs attained a higher degree in nursing (51.9 per cent receiving a B.S., 47.5 per cent a master's, and 0.6 per cent a doctorate) (6, Table II-C-4). The nursing labor force as a whole is heavily concentrated, in terms of educational credentials, at the lower degree levels. Thus in 1972, of 778,470 employed RNs in the U.S., 80.5 per cent had less than a B.A. or B.S.; 14.3 per cent had attained a bachelor's degree; 3.2 per cent held a master's degree; and 0.2 per cent held a doctorate (6, Table I-A-3).

Two-thirds of the RNs with A.D.s or diplomas worked in hospitals, as did 56 per cent of those with baccalaureate degrees and 32 per cent of those with higher degrees. In the hospitals, the latter groups tended to occupy the supervisory and administrative positions. It is in the hospitals, which have become the typical workplaces for the nursing labor force, where we see the hierarchical division of labor between all types of nursing workers, RNs, PNs, and NAs, most vividly.

The Nursing Hierarchy

The average hospital in the U.S. is a large bureaucratic enterprise (7); that is, a workplace which is characterized by impersonal work relations, a highly specialized division of labor, and clearly delineated levels of authority. In 1972, there were 7,061 hospitals in the U.S. with 1,549,665 beds, or an average of 219.5 beds per hospital. The nursing service departments of these hospitals employed an average (in "full-time equivalents") per hospital of 79 NAs, 35 PNs, and 61 RNs. ("Full-time equivalents" are calculated under the assumption that the average part-time worker is a half-time worker.)

The NAs are on the bottom in terms of hierarchical authority and control. According to the American Nurses Association, the role of the nursing aide

> ... is that of assisting the RN or LPN (licensed practical nurse) in the nursing service, which operates according to the type of health facility it serves. This work is delegated by an RN and performed under the direction of an RN or LPN. It consists of simple tasks involved in assisting in the personal care of individuals who are ill or otherwise disabled and assisting in the maintenance of a safe and healthful environment (8; see also 9, p. 216; 10).

Next up the ladder comes the practical nurse who provides "nursing care and treatment of patients under the supervision of a licensed physician or registered nurse.... They may also assist with the supervision of nursing aides, orderlies and attendants" (5, p. 216; see also 10).

Among the RNs, the lowest level of the hierarchy is occupied by the general duty or staff nurse. While she/he may give orders to NAs and PNs, she/he may also find herself/himself doing the same type of tasks as these other workers. These staff nurses belong to nursing units which are supervised by head nurses and their assistants, who in turn are directed and evaluated by supervisors of nurses and their assistants. The hierarchical arrangement from the nursing aides to the supervisors of nurses constitutes the inpatient nursing service of the hospital. All these nursing workers are directly or indirectly responsible to the director of nursing, who also presides over the administrative nursing unit (consisting of nursing instructors, consultants, and other administrative personnel). All these nursing workers, including the director of nursing, are under the direction of the doctors and administrators who control the hospital.

Table 2 shows the quantitative dimensions of this hierarchy in the "average" hospital. (Here, as elsewhere, the average includes hospitals of various sizes and types. For more specific purposes of analyses, hospitals should be disaggregated by size and function.) In this table we have also indicated the distribution of male RNs in the RN hierarchy. Although men constituted only 1.7 per cent of RNs in hospitals in 1972, they were disproportionately distributed in the administrative and supervisory (as well as other special) roles.

The Structure of Wages

We can also demonstrate the extent of this hierarchy in quantitative terms by the relative wages paid to different sectors of the nursing labor force. In Table 3 we show the structure of wages in August 1972 in nonfederal hospitals in five representative cities selected from different parts of the United States. (In 1971, nongovernment hospitals were 63.5 per cent of all hospitals, while 31.1 per cent were state and local government hospitals and 5.3 per cent were federal hospitals. Of the nongovernment hospitals, 21.8 per cent were proprietary hospitals and 78.2 per cent were "nonprofit" hospitals) (5, p. 369).

Public health nursing workers have a hierarchical structure of wages similar to that of hospital nursing workers: the median wage of higher-level RNs is up to three times that of public health assistants and home health aides, with staff RNs occupying an intermediary position in the wage structure (11).

Table 2

Distribution of registered nurses in the U.S. hospital nursing labor force,
by sex and position in the hospital hierarchy, in 1972[a]

Category	Nursing Workers	Per cent of All RNs	Male RNs	Per cent of All Male RNs	Nursing Workers per Hospital[b]
Registered nurses	499,594	100.0	8646	100.0	61.10
Administration					
Director or					
assistant	13,953	2.8	568	6.6	1.91
Consultant	2,079	0.4	46	0.5	0.28
Instructor	7,150	1.4	194	2.2	0.96
Inpatient care					
Supervisor or					
assistant	54,445	10.9	1453	16.8	7.29
Head nurse or					
assistant	89,952	18.0	1452	16.8	12.23
Staff nurse	309,794	62.0	2893	33.5	35.54
Other specified					
type	11,290	2.3	1697	19.6	1.47
Not reported	10,931	2.2	343	4.0	1.42
Practical nurses	270,000				35.18
Nursing aides,					
orderlies, and					
attendants	597,000				79.48

[a]Source, reference 6, Tables I-A-6, I-A-9, IV-A-1, IV-B-1.
[b]Full-time equivalents.

Female RNs working in nonsupervisory positions in occupational health tend to earn somewhat less than general duty nurses in hospitals. In February 1972, the average weekly salary of occupational health nurses in the U.S. was $169.00 ($196.50 in the northeast, $161.50 in the south, $173.50 in the north central region, and $179.00 in the west) (6, Table III-D-2). The minimum 8-hour fees for private duty nurses (as established by State Nurses Associations) ranged, in January 1973, from $28.00 in Alabama to $43.00 in Pennsylvania (or from $140.00 to $215.00 for a standard 40-hour week, although it must be recognized that private duty employment is much more irregular than employment in other types of nursing) (6, p. 129).

When educational credentials, skills, and responsibility are taken into consideration, nursing workers in general are poorly paid relative to other occupational groups in the U.S. economy, as illustrated in Table 4.

From what we have presented thus far, it is evident that while some of the nurses at the top of the nursing hierarchy are relatively well paid and have some control over the day-to-day functioning of the work process, the vast majority of nursing workers receive relatively low wages and have little control over the use of their own labor or the product of their labor. And however much the incomes *within* the nursing labor force vary, these differentials are small compared with those between doctors, on the one hand, and nursing workers in general, on the other.

In 1972, there were 356,384 doctors of medicine in the U.S. Of these, 333,259 were active in the practice of medicine. However, only 269,095 (or 80.7 per cent of active doctors) actually provided patient care to civilians, that is, one MD for every

Table 3

Wage structure of RNs (female), PNs (female), and NAs in nonfederal hospitals by selected metropolitan areas, August 1972 (for standard 39.5- to 40-hour work week)[a]

Category	Atlanta Wage	Atlanta Index[b]	Boston Wage	Boston Index	Chicago Wage	Chicago Index	Dallas Wage	Dallas Index	S.F.–Oakland Wage	S.F.–Oakland Index
Nongovernment hospitals										
Director of nursing	$292.50	175.1	$346.00	188.0	$329.00	178.3	$242.00	147.1	$325.00	154.0
Supervisor of nurses	199.50	119.5	241.50	131.0	236.00	127.9	199.00	121.0	257.00	121.8
Nursing instructor	173.00	103.6	229.50	124.7	226.00	122.5	215.00	130.7	248.00	117.5
Head nurse	188.00	112.6	218.50	118.8	217.00	117.6	184.00	111.9	236.50	112.1
General duty nurse	167.00	100.0	184.00	100.0	184.50	100.0	164.50	100.0	211.00	100.0
Practical nurse	119.50	71.6	148.00	80.4	145.00	78.6	107.50	65.0	165.00	78.2
Nursing aide (female)	94.50	56.6	108.50	59.0	115.50	62.6	82.50	50.2	145.00	68.7
Nursing aide (male)	96.50	57.8	113.00	61.4	113.00	61.6	87.50	53.2	145.00	68.7
Nonfederal government hospitals										
Director of nursing	$310.00	177.1	$304.00	161.7	$388.00	194.5	$ n.a.[c]	—	$372.00	170.6
Supervisor of nurses	216.00	123.4	243.50	129.5	265.00	132.8	228.50	135.6	283.50	130.0
Nursing instructor	203.00	116.0	246.50	131.1	229.00	114.8	n.a.	—	286.50	131.4
Head nurse	192.50	110.0	221.50	117.8	231.50	116.0	197.00	116.9	257.00	117.9
General duty nurse	175.00	100.0	188.00	100.0	199.50	100.0	168.50	100.0	218.00	100.0
Practical nurse	123.00	70.0	153.00	81.4	153.50	76.9	122.50	72.7	164.00	75.2
Nursing aide (female)	93.00	53.1	123.50	65.7	136.00	68.2	96.50	57.3	150.00	68.8
Nursing aide (male)	93.50	53.4	119.00	63.3	132.50	66.4	n.a.	—	151.00	69.3

[a]Source, reference 6, Tables III-B-3, III-B-4, IV-D-1, IV-D-4.
[b]Average earnings of general duty nurse = 100.
[c]n.a. signifies data not available.

Table 4

Median earnings of fully employed (50-52 weeks) females in
selected occupational categories, 1969[a]

Category	Earnings
Secondary school teachers	$7534
Social and recreation workers	7241
Elementary school and kindergarten teachers	7097
Registered nurses	6807
Health technologists and technicians	5985
Secretaries	5681
Office machine operators	5240
Telephone operators	5121
Practical nurses	4919
Operatives (except transport)	4334
Hairdressers and cosmetologists	3900
Nursing aides and attendants	3681
Cleaning service workers	3465
Food service workers	2823

[a]Source, U.S. Bureau of the Census. *1970 Census of the Population: Detailed Characteristics*, pp. 1-772, 1-773. U.S. Government Printing Office, Washington, D.C., 1971.

780 people in the U.S. civilian population (6, Tables V-B-1, V-B-2). The average income of MDs was, in 1972, about $46,500 or about 2.5-3 times the average salary of a director of nursing and 5 times the average salary of the general duty nurse.

Nursing Workers and Doctors

In 1972, with about 269,000 doctors and 705,000 nurses providing patient care, the ratio of MDs to RNs delivering direct health care (i.e. nonadministrative doctors and nurses) was 1 to 2.6. The ratio of MDs to all nursing workers providing patient care (1,962,000) for 1972 was 1 to 7.3. The ratio of total active MDs (federal and nonfederal, practice, research, and administrative) to the total nursing labor force in 1972 was 1 to 6.1.

Of course, these aggregate statistics do not reveal the great concentration of nursing workers in hospitals nor do they reveal the disparities of power and income among doctors (e.g. that one-fifth of all active doctors in 1972 were interns and residents in hospitals, and that a large proportion of the less desirable medical positions were occupied by the approximately 15 per cent of the U.S. physicians who were from foreign, and especially Third World, countries) (12). However, the general importance of the nursing labor force to the power and income of doctors and hospitals in the 1970s becomes evident when it is considered that in 1900, there were about 131,000 physicians in the U.S., or one MD for every 577 people, about 11,000 graduate nurses (13, p. 37), and approximately 109,000 "untrained" or "practical" nurses (including midwives), and hence less than one nursing worker for every doctor. Underlying the changes in these quantitative dimensions from 1900 to the present, there is the story of the integration of the nursing work force into the health industry as the wage-laborers for doctors and hospitals.

THE INTEGRATION OF THE NURSING LABOR FORCE
INTO THE HEALTH INDUSTRY

19th-Century Nursing

Throughout most of the 19th century, there was no organized nursing labor force in the United States. There were no schools of nursing nor was there any systematic public (or private) control over the quality and quantity of nurses. As late as 1860, 80 per cent of the people in the U.S. still lived in rural areas. By this time, however, cities, and the general population, were expanding rapidly. By 1900 the proportion of the people living in rural areas had declined to 60 per cent but in absolute numbers the rural inhabitants had risen by over 80 per cent since 1860 (14, p. 9). In rural areas, nursing (i.e. bedside care) was performed on an informal basis by members of the local community, while in the large cities some hospitals were set up by religious orders and charitable organizations. Many of these hospitals were originally established as alms houses—health care delivery to the urban poor was considered charity in this period (15). In 1848, The Bellevue Hospital in New York opened as the first institution to be entirely devoted to the care of the sick (15, p. 288; 16).

The lack of organization in nursing care reflected the lack of organization in health care delivery in general (17). By the outbreak of the Civil War some beginnings were being made in the training of nurses by women physicians who were interested in providing women with better obstetrical and gynecological care. The Women's Medical College in Philadelphia started a nursing school in 1861 as had the New England Female (Medical) College in 1860. The New England Hospital for Women and Children trained 30 nurses between 1862 and 1872 (15). At this time, however, most maternity care was delivered by midwives who carried out their practice independent of doctors.

The Civil War brought on a need for a large number of people to render aid in military hospitals, both in giving direct assistance to doctors and in maintaining the hospitals and patients in something approaching a state of sanitation. An estimated 2,000 nurses participated in the Civil War (18, p. 183). Numerous untrained women volunteered as nurses but it was certainly not a "women's" occupation—male nurses or orderlies outnumbered women in military wards by 2 to 1 (15).

The main enduring effect of the Civil War on the development of a nursing labor force was that it put some women in positions of leadership and gave them experience in training nurses and organizing health teams (15). For example, Elizabeth Blackwell, the first woman physician in the U.S., had trained 100 Union nurses during the Civil War. After the war, some of these women sought to accommodate a growing demand for nurses as urban areas grew and as the growing number of medical doctors looked to nurses as a way of expanding "their" delivery of health service. The new supplies of nurses came from two sources. First, there were the upper-class women in the cities who took an interest in urban reform and who set out to organize nursing in the last decades of the 19th century. Following the model that Florence Nightingale had set out in England (19), these women (who were usually unmarried) established in the 1870s and 1880s the first of the modern-type schools of nursing (i.e. schools where graduate nurses taught student nurses). At schools such as Bellevue and Johns Hopkins attempts were made to attract upper-class women by putting forth nursing as a socially useful alternative to motherhood (17). But as the need for nurses expanded toward the end of the century, the actual women who did the nursing came from another source: working-class women who were not looking to nursing primarily as a means of performing their "feminine" role in society, but rather primarily because they had to work to earn a living.

Growth of Nursing Schools

In 1880, there were 15 nursing schools with 323 students in the United States. By 1890, these numbers had grown to 35 schools with 1,552 students. The number of graduate nurses available to teach facilitated the increase and expansion of these schools. There were 225 nursing schools by 1893, and 432 (training 11,164 nurses and graduating 3,500) in 1900. It was not, however, the supply of teaching nurses but rather the labor needs of hospitals which brought the nursing schools into existence in the last decade of the 19th century. Hospitals were undergoing a rapid expansion at this time. Statistics on the number of hospitals in the U.S. are not available for this period. However, we do know that in 1873, there were 178 hospitals with 34,453 beds in the U.S., and by 1909 there were 4,359 hospitals with 421,065 beds (14, Series B235-238; 15; 20, p. 83). From the 1870s the largest nursing schools, such as Bellevue, New Haven, and Massachusetts General, had been part of hospitals. During the 1870s and 1880s, many nursing schools which had tried to function independently of hospitals found themselves in continuing financial difficulties, and either died out or merged with the hospitals. The hospitals were willing to finance these schools, and also to establish new schools, in return for the right to use the labor of the student nurses in their wards as well as in "private duty" service in the homes of the patrons of the hospitals. As a leading nursing educator wrote in the early 1890s, "Practically, then, the hospital secures nursing for $12 a month on its payroll, which at its market value would bring at least $15 a week ..." (21). From this time to the 1930s, student nurses provided the main labor force for hospitals.

With the integration of nursing schools into hospitals, a great deal of control over nursing passed out of the hands of even the elite of the nursing labor force (21). First, the actual training of student nurses often took second place to the performance of routine hospital services by these students. Second, the hospital superintendents of nursing (nurses, usually female) did not have ultimate control over the development of nurse training, but rather were responsible to the director of the hospital (almost always a male). This lack of control was put quite plainly by Josephine Goldmark in her influential report in 1923. While being careful not to attack the hospital hierarchy, she voiced the following complaint (22, p. 205):

> The hospital superintendent is an expert along many lines, but in most instances he is not an educator. Yet he is practically in control of the pedagogical methods of what purports to be an educational institution. Generally the superintendent of the hospital appoints, or, what amounts to the same thing, recommends for appointment, the superintendent of nurses. In most cases his power of veto or of approval over the policies of the training school is absolute, for it is only through him that the head of the training school has any access to the final authorities, the hospital trustees. Finally, he is usually a physician; she a nurse. The etiquette of the profession, discipline, and the hard-worked plea of "loyalty" to the institution effectually prevent any direct appeal to the hospital board.

Nursing Organizations

In the 1890s, however, the nursing elite did try to organize themselves so as to exert some control over the development of their "profession." (If we define a professional occupation not only as one involving high levels of technical skills and complex mental processes, but also one where the practitioners maintain autonomy over both their work and the development of their skills, then nursing lost out on any professional status it might have had when the nursing schools became integrated into the hospital setting.) In 1893, 20 superintendents of these nursing schools met at the International Congress of Charities, Correction, and Philanthropy in Chicago. The following year they formed the American Society of Superintendents of Training Schools for Nurses of the U.S. and Canada. In 1912 this organization was renamed the National League of Nursing Education, which (as the National League of Nursing) remains the primary organ of the American Nurses Association (ANA) for nurse control over nurse education.

In 1894 a "professional" organization was formed for the graduate nurses in general called the Nurses Associated Alumnae of the United States and Canada. In 1911 this group was renamed the American Nurses Association (15).

These organizations, however, sought their power and occupational status in a health sector run by doctors. At the same time, many if not most nurses practiced independently of doctors as private duty nurses in homes and in community agencies (23). In addition, "nurses" performed one of the most necessary medical functions—obstetrics. As late as 1910, 50 per cent of all babies in the U.S. were delivered by midwives working independently of doctors (17). (It is difficult to estimate the number of midwives at that time. In the statistics available, they are lumped together with "practical" nurses, who were called "untrained" nurses by the nursing "profession.") In 1880 there were an estimated 13,485 practical nurses including midwives in the U.S.; in 1890, 42,586; in 1900, 103,747; and in 1910, 126,836 (24, p. 28). As the medical profession consolidated its power after the Flexner Report in 1910, midwifery was outlawed in many states with the exception of rural and slightly populated areas where doctors did not desire to practice. As doctors institutionalized the hierarchical division of labor between their own numbers and nurses, graduate nurses sought to achieve economic security and occupational status by legislating standards for the education and employment of nurses. In its report in 1899, the Nurses Associated Alumnae stated the main problem which was to confront nurses in the coming decades: "The country has been flooded with a very nondescript class of women, all bearing the title of trained nurse, the term standing for all grades of training and all grades of women" (25, p. 139). In 1900, this organization started the *American Journal of Nursing,* which pushed registration of nurses as a means for controlling and upgrading the occupation, arguing that nurses, like doctors, should be legally licensed. The first registration law was passed (20, p. 152) in North Carolina in 1903 and, despite the opposition of hospitals and businesses offering short courses and correspondence courses in nursing, by 1917 45 states and two territories of the United States had followed suit (6, p. 60-62). RNs sat on the state boards and set schooling and practice standards.

Controlling the Supply of Doctors: The Flexner Report

Meanwhile, the medical profession was consolidating its own power as a dominating force in the health care sector. In 1904, the American Medical Association (AMA) Council on Medical Education began to classify medical schools in an attempt to control the expansion of the supply of physicians (14, p. 31). With the help of the Carnegie Corporation, and through the instrument of the Flexner Report, begun in 1907 and finished in 1910, the AMA managed to gain unchallenged control over medical education, and hence over the quantity and quality of members of their own profession. Taking the Johns Hopkins Medical School as his model, Flexner surveyed the existing medical schools and ordered them to adapt to Hopkins' standards or close. At the same time he recommended that the number of medical schools be reduced from 155 to 31, and even included a map in his report showing the location of the schools destined to survive (26). He argued that there were too many doctors in the United States and that the total number of graduates should be reduced from 4,442 (in 1910) to about 2,000 annually and that the number should then be allowed to rise in proportion to the increase in the nation's population. There was no attempt to direct some of the resources of the Carnegie Corporation toward upgrading the less-well-endowed schools such as the medical schools for blacks and women. Rather, those schools which were deemed unfit were pressured into closing (27, 28).

The Flexner proposals were instituted quite effectively as can be clearly seen in Table 5. By 1929 only one "unapproved" school remained (14, p. 31).

Table 5

Medical schools and the supply of physicians, 1900–1929[a]

Year	Medical Schools	Students	Graduates	Physicians[b]	Physicians per 100,000 Population
1900	160	25,171	5,214	119,749	157
1906	162	25,204	5,364	134,688	158
1909	151	22,602	4,741	134,402	149
1910	131	21,526	4,440	135,000	146
1912	118	18,482	4,483	137,199	144
1914	102	16,502	3,594	142,332	144
1916	95	14,012	3,518	145,241	142
1918	90	13,630	2,670	147,812	141
1921	83	14,466	3,186	145,404	134
1923	80	16,960	3,120	145,966	130
1925	80	18,200	3,974	147,010	127
1929	76	20,878	4,446	152,503	125

[a]Source, reference 14, Series B 180-181, 186-188.
[b]Includes inactive physicians and those in federal service.

Supply of Nurses Expands

While the nursing registration laws did give the graduate nursing bodies some control over the standards of nursing education and practice, they did not, in contrast to the case of the AMA, give them the power to restrict the number of schools or to outlaw the practice of nursing by those not trained in their schools. Hence, they did not secure control of the quantitative development of the trained and untrained nursing labor supplies. The number of nursing schools and the number of trained nurses expanded rapidly in the first three decades of the 20th century, as shown in Table 6.

Table 6

Nursing schools and the supply of registered nurses 1900–1929[a]

Year	Nursing Schools	Students	Graduates	Active RNs	Active RNs/MDs
1900	432	11,164	3,465	11,804[b]	0.10
1905	862	19,824	5,795		
1910	1,129	32,636	8,140	50,500	0.37
1915	1,509	46,141	11,116		
1920	1,755	54,958	14,980	103,900	0.72
1927	1,797	77,768	18,628		
1929	1,885	78,771	23,810	214,300[c]	1.39[c]

[a]Source, reference 14, Series B 180, 184-185, 192-194.
[b]May include some students.
[c]1930 figures.

Most nurses continued to care for patients in their homes, either through a doctor or through a nursing registry. Registries were set up by nursing schools, district nursing associations, and individuals as central employment bureaus for nurses. By World War I, all the major nursing schools had registries (20, Ch. 6). A survey of over 24,000 RNs taken in 1927 by the Committee on the Grading of Nursing Schools showed that 54 per cent were in private duty nursing, 19 per cent were in public health nursing, and 23 per cent in institutional work (4 per cent were in unclassified activities) (13, p. 249). According to one estimate 69 per cent of graduating nurses in 1928 went into private duty nursing (20, Ch. 5).

Public health nursing was a product of the first decades of the 20th century. In the 1880s, visiting nurse associations had been formed in the big cities as a form of charitable work (15). By 1901 there were 130 of these "visiting" or public health nurses; by 1914, 5,152; by 1919, 8,770; and by 1923, 11,000 (22, p. 42). The development of the public health movement and of this type of nurse was in response to the sanitation problems in the rapidly growing urban areas in this period. However, much of the resources for the employment of these nurses came from a new source. In 1909, the Metropolitan Life Insurance Company started a successful experiment in sending public health nurses into the homes of its policy holders for the purpose of lowering the mortality rates among its clients and hence saving on death claims. By the early 1920s, Metropolitan was employing 500 nurses directly and had working agreements with 650 visiting nurse associations in 2,000 cities. The company estimated that in 1920 alone it saved $4.7 million on death claims by expending $1.4 million on visiting nurses and general welfare work for its own policy holders (20, p. 157; 22, p. 52).

In 1920, only 11,000 out of almost 104,000 RNs (not including nursing students) in the U.S. were working in hospitals and other institutions (22, p. 17). It is possible that this number declined during the 1920s, for we have another estimate of 4,000 RNs in hospitals in 1929 (29). In any case, Goldmark devoted only one page of her 580-page report specifically to institutional nursing, as opposed to public health and private duty nursing, explaining that it did not require separate treatment (22, p. 184). Many hospitals found their labor supplies in the 54,953 students in the nursing schools. Hospitals without schools often used untrained or "practical" nurses who were significantly cheaper than trained nurses. (This was especially true of the 521 mental hospitals which contained 36 per cent of the total hospital beds in the U.S. in 1920. General hospitals were still relatively small, averaging 78 beds (14, pp. 209-220).) The supply of these untrained nurses had been growing steadily from 133,043 in 1910 to 156,767 in 1920 (hence untrained nurses still outnumbered trained nurses by 3 to 2).

Controlling the Nursing Work Force: The Goldmark Report

The numbers of PNs and RNs had rapidly increased during World War I (25, pp. 190, 195). In 1918, the use of paid aides was started in hospitals (20, Ch. 6). After the war there was an abundant supply of cheap nursing labor. In addition, numerous commercial short-courses had been set up to supply the nursing needs created by both the war and the flu epidemic of 1918. Those profiting from these courses tried to continue to expand the supply of nurses after the war. In this they were aided by a proliferation of new hospitals, mostly proprietary and quite small, which were ready to hire any cheap nursing labor (25, pp. 193-194). By 1924, there were more hospitals in the United States than there are today, the number having grown from 5,323 in 1918 to 7,370 in 1924. In the latter year, 2,397 hospitals were proprietary (with an average of 29.9 beds per hospital), the number of these hospitals having increased by 36 per cent since 1923 (14, Series B235-248).

In the face of this situation, a committee, made up of physicians (mostly related to prestigious medical schools and all male) as well as RNs and other women, was formed between 1918 and 1920 (22, p. v). Under the auspices of the Rockefeller Foundation, this committee set out to investigate nursing and nursing education in the U.S. The findings of this committee received a great deal of publicity when they were issued, in 1923, under the popular name of the Goldmark Report (25, p. 203).

The main problem confronting the development of the nursing labor supply was clearly stated by Goldmark in this report:

> With the unquestioned tendency of newly trained subsidiary workers to disperse after graduation and the impossibility of gauging the competence or training of those already working independently, we are forced to query what procedure shall be advocated to fill the unquestionable need for bedside attendants in large numbers, while safeguarding on the one hand the patients whose lives and comfort may be jeopardized by incompetence, and safeguarding on the other hand the hard won status and guarantee of the R.N. (22, p. 177).

The committee made two very specific proposals to handle this problem:

1. That steps should be taken through state legislation for the definition and licensure of a subsidiary grade of nursing service, the subsidiary type of worker to serve under practicing physicians in the care of mild and chronic illness, and convalescence, and possibly to assist under the direction of the trained nurse in certain phases of hospital and visiting nursing.
2. That when the licensure of a subsidiary grade of nursing service is provided for, the establishment of training courses in preparation for such service is highly desirable; that such courses should be conducted in special hospitals, or in separate sections of hospitals where nurses are also trained; and that the course should be of eight or nine weeks' duration; provided the standards of such schools be approved by the same educational board which governs nursing training schools (22, pp. 16, 28).

To avoid confusion by patients and doctors as to what they were really getting when they hired practical nurses at $25 per week rather than registered nurses at $35 per week, the committee recommended that the commonly used term "practical nurse" be dropped, and that the "subsidiary workers" be called "nursing aides" or "nursing attendants." They also recommended that the public should be educated as to the difference between these two types of nurses. Hence, there would be no question in the minds of the public or employers that a "nurse" is a professional, registered nurse (22, p. 16).

The committee also sought to standardize the training of "graduate" nurses, extend the principle of registration to all these nurses, and legitimize their higher wages. In this area, the main problem confronting the committee was the fact that the development of trained nurses had since the 1890s been dependent on direct financing from hospitals which in return were assured of a relatively cheap, and often more tractable, labor supply (13, pp. 410-416, 434-438). The committee wanted to put an end to this situation by substituting for student labor that of "nursing aides." The training period for "professional" nurses would now be reduced from the usual 3 years to 28 months. Training time would be saved without any sacrifice of educational quality by "the elimination of unrewarding routine service" (22, p. 22).

In addition, the committee proposed that control over hospital education be taken out of the hands of the hospitals and put into the hands of educators affiliated with schools of nursing at universities. They saw this as a way of bypassing responsibility to the boards of trustees of hospitals, as well as a way of attracting more independent financial support for nursing and elevating the status of the profession. Their intention was that the actual university schools would train the elite of the nursing profession. From this elite would come the administrators and teachers who would be in charge of training regular nurses in hospital schools while remaining responsible to the university schools. "The university school of nursing," they envisaged, "would be the keystone of the whole arch."

> It will not only train leaders and develop and standardize procedures for all other schools. It will, by its permeating influence, give inspiration and balance to the movement as a whole and gradually but steadily improve the efficiency of every institution for the training of nurses of whatever type (22, p. 26).

These proposals did not meet with the immediate acceptance of doctors and hospital administrators. Goldmark herself recognized the opposition that attempts to upgrade nurses would receive from physicians. As she stated in her report:

> We have the extreme view expressed by many physicians that for bedside care the present nurse is "over-trained"; that her charges are so exorbitant as to be prohibitive for all but the very rich; that the nurse is merely the doctor's "extended hands"; hence, that any biddable girl can be quickly trained to obtain the necessary deftness and skill to carry out his orders.

But Goldmark was quick to add, "It is of course true that a leading element of the medical profession does not share these views" (22, p. 162).

However, the proposals, because they did not challenge the right to rule of the physicians and hospital administrators over the health sector and because, in fact, they sought to take into account the labor supply needs of doctors and hospitals, were to have long-run significance as a model both for stratification within the ranks of registered nurses and for the protection of registered nurses in general from an expanded supply of "subsidiary workers."

Economic Depression Takes Control

However, the main changes in the character of nursing and nursing education which were to take place in the period between the Goldmark Report and World War II were due not so much to the conscious efforts of the nursing and medical elites to rationalize the supply of nurses as to the changing economic pressures on nurses as the U.S. economy passed from prosperity to depression. In 1928, employment conditions for graduate nurses were already "extremely bad" (13, p. 83) due to the rapid and uncontrolled expansion of their numbers since World War I. The situation for nurses therefore became all the more serious when the depression hit the U.S. economy at the end of 1929 (25, p. 239). Unemployment and falling levels of income forced many Americans to cut drastically their expenditures on health care (precisely at the time when they needed such services most). Especially cut back was the use of private duty nurses in homes. The ANA was, at first, reluctant to use what power it had to ease the plight of nurses. For example, at the beginning of the depression, the ANA resisted the substitution of an 8-hour day for RNs for the usual 12-hour day (which would have allowed more nurses to share the limited amount of work) on the grounds that, as professionals, their workday was dictated by the needs of the patients for service (20, Ch. 5). The ANA did set up a relief fund for unemployed nurses but this was very quickly depleted by payments to nurses who had contracted tuberculosis while at work (25, pp. 191-192). However, as the depression deepened, the ANA came around to supporting an 8-hour day, share-the-work plan (25, pp. 191-192).

Meanwhile, during the depression years of the 1930s, the number of nursing schools was rapidly decreasing. With the oversupply of nursing labor, the National League of Nursing Education had a sound economic basis for putting into effect the higher minimum standards for nursing schools for which it had been pushing since the Goldmark Report. At the same time, the task of establishing these standards by eliminating the low-grade nursing schools was made possible by the fact that many smaller hospitals were voluntarily closing their nursing schools. With so many graduate nurses unemployed, it was now cheaper for the hospital to hire them, often for little more than room and board, than to operate the nursing school as its primary source of labor (20, pp. 193-194). From 1929 to 1940, the number of RN schools decreased from 1,885 to 1,311, with most of the decline in the first half of the decade. Those that remained became larger, the average number of students per school rising from 42 in 1929 to 65 in 1940 (14, Series B192-194).

Shift to Hospital Nursing

As a longer-run phenomenon, the use of graduate nurses (and other full-time nursing workers) instead of student nurses as the primary labor force in the hospital had its origins during the 1930s when health care delivery in general shifted from the family home to the hospital. Childbirths, for example, moved from the home to the hospital in the 1930s (20, p. 195). The change was partly due to the development of capital-intensive medical techniques which had to be housed in a central location (20, pp. 194-196). But perhaps more important in this respect was the development of hospital insurance. During the early 1930s, with hospitals suffering from lack of paying patients, hospital insurance groups were started in order to spread the costs of medical care among a wider population than those who would actually utilize the hospitals, and hence generate a demand for hospital services which most individuals could not have otherwise afforded. In 1934, there were 100,000 subscribers to hospital insurance plans and by 1936, 450,000. Under the symbol of the Blue Cross the number of subscribers reached 1,500,000 by 1938 and 6,049,222 by 1941 (20, p. 197; 30, p. 23).

As a result of the growing predominance of the hospital in health care delivery and the decline in the number of hospital schools, the number of graduate nurses employed in hospitals rose sharply, according to one estimate from 4,000 in 1929 to 28,000 in 1937 (29). By the end of the decade institutional nursing had replaced private duty nursing as the top employment category for nurses (with public health nursing third).

Consolidation of the Nursing Hierarchy

The private duty RN had seen the private duty PN as a price-cutting competitor on the labor market. The competitive market relation did not disappear with the shift to hospital work. But now the relation between the RN and the PN was more than one of two isolated workers competing for a job. Now they were expected to work together to deliver health care in the hospital setting. The impersonal market relation between the two workers had become a concrete social relation in the labor process. While the administrators had an interest in maintaining some degree of competitive tension between these workers, this tension had to be mitigated to some extent to permit a cooperative work effort to take place. One way for the hospitals to resolve this contradiction was to clearly demarcate lines of authority and job functions between these two classifications of workers while at the same time retaining the right to change the organization of work when the situation called for it (e.g. when the hospital administrators felt that they could get away with shifting an RN job function onto a cheaper labor supply). Hence, while the two groups of workers would cooperate on the job, the RNs, despite their hierarchical position, would always feel threatened by the very existence of the PNs, while the PNs would feel cut off from the RNs by the lines of authority.

The ANA aided the hospitals in this process of rationalizing the hierarchy as it began to look more closely at ways to protect the job status of the RNs from the threat posed by these "auxiliary" or "subsidiary" workers (25, p. 248). One form of control was the licensure of practical nurses (31), with RNs supervising the state licensing boards and setting educational standards and employment criteria in such a way so as to clearly draw the line between the PN and RN (18, p. 321; 24, Ch. 13-16). As one authority on PNs (herself an RN) wrote:

> Overtraining can be a serious danger. The practical nurse who has a course of over fifteen months (theory and practice) gets a false impression of her abilities and builds up the unwarranted belief that she can practice as a professional nurse (24, p. 261).

With the backing of the ANA, the licensure of PNs went forward at a rapid pace after World War II, until by 1955 all the states and some of the territories of the U.S. had licensing boards (32).

The 1940s also saw a great expansion in a third category of nursing workers— nursing aides (including attendants and orderlies). In 1940, there were approximately 102,000 nursing aides employed in the U.S. The supply of these personnel was expanded with the assistance of the American Red Cross which, in 1938, had started a program (10 weeks in duration) to train nursing aides in hospitals. By 1945, 212,000 women had been certified as nursing aides through these programs (9, p. 16). By 1950, there were 216,000 nursing aides, attendants, and orderlies employed in the U.S., virtually all of whom were working in hospitals and nursing homes. A quote from an influential 1948 report on nursing by Brown (33) tells much of the story of the integration of nursing aides into the health team of the general hospital:

> No one assumes that the task of creating efficient, differentiated but integrated nursing service based upon functional requisites will be easy or readily accomplished, or that progress will everywhere be uniform. . . . How various kinds of personnel can be better selected and trained, and their efforts coordinated is the problem to be solved. Particularly instructive is an experiment now being undertaken in one large general hospital in solving the problem of unsatisfactory ward attendants. This hospital had been much impressed by the intelligence, understanding, and interest shown by the nurse's aides who had volunteered their services during the war. Could personnel be found and trained to replace the attendants, who would more nearly resemble these former volunteers? Public announcement was made of raised standards for application and improved wages. In response to this request for persons designated as nursing aides, the hospital discovered among the large Negro community a hitherto untapped reservoir of personnel, well above the ward attendant group in intelligence and personality.

Also in 1948, Eli Ginzberg, then chairman of the Committee on the Functions of Nursing, put forth a general principle of economics to be applied by employers in the health industry: "Never use high-priced personnel for low-priced work" (quoted in 9, p. 27). In the next section we will discuss the broader implications of this approach to the operation of the health care industry, especially as it applies to the development of nursing labor supplies.

THE NURSING LABOR FORCE AND
THE HEALTH INDUSTRY SINCE THE 1940s

Rationalization of the Nursing Hierarchy

By the late 1940s, the general structure of the nursing labor force as it now exists had clearly taken shape. The hospital had become the primary workplace of the nursing labor force, and the major divisions among nursing workers had been institutionalized by means of educational standards, licensure, job descriptions, and the formation of various occupational organizations. Within the context of this general structure, the specifics of the hierarchical division of labor remained, and still remain, very much in flux. As stated in a report on a series of nursing studies made between 1951 and 1957 (34):

> To generalize broadly from the reports today, the professional nurse is chiefly an administrator, organizer and teacher, and the practical nurse is the bedside tender. More accurately this is a statement of trends. What is a fait accompli in some hospitals is the coming thing in others; the frontiers of work of the various ranks of nurses are shifting lines and the sifting and sorting of tasks is still going on in hospitals all over the country; but it was not planned or foreseen and it proceeds at an uneven pace, differing from one hospital to another, uncontrolled and unpredictable. . . . Study after study corroborates the chief point: that today not one but several categories of nurse attend the sick and run the hospitals and that the frontiers of each one's work are all changing at once.

Since the 1950s, the functions of the different types of nursing workers have been continuously defined and redefined. With the rise of a variety of "allied health professions," many tasks previously performed by RNs are now undertaken by other health workers (31, 35). In many cases, however, the boundaries of occupational responsibilities have been left purposely ambiguous by hospital administrators to permit a certain amount of flexibility in the allocation of day-to-day tasks among the existing labor supply.

But despite all the changes in work organization in the health industry over the past 25 years, the broad separation of the nursing labor force into RNs, PNs, and NAs still prevails. In what follows we will abstract from the particular ways in which the division of labor in the health industry has taken place in order to focus on the more general changes in the development of the nursing labor force over the past 25 years. Then we will discuss the general implications of these changes for the role of the nursing work force in movements to restructure the health industry.

Expansion of Hospital Nursing

Table 7 shows the quantitative development of the nursing labor force employed in hospitals. As can be seen from this table, the numbers of all categories of the nursing labor force have expanded greatly since 1950. However, the rate of growth of the number of PNs has been especially rapid, and this group has become a very important sector of the hospital nursing labor force.

Women's Work and Women Workers

It should be noted that this expansion of the nursing labor force in the hospital setting has not led to any "defeminization" of registered nurses. In 1950, 97.6 per cent

Table 7

Registered nurses, practical nurses, and nursing aides in the nursing labor force in the United States, 1950–1972[a]

Year	Numbers Employed in Hospitals			Per cent of Total Nursing Labor Force Employed in Hospitals		
	RNs	PNs	NAs	RNs	PNs	NAs
1950	238,128	42,000[b]	228,819[b]	46.8	8.3	45.0
1956	265,800	70,758	281,560	43.0	11.4	45.5
1960	320,000	107,000[c]	366,000[c]	40.3	13.5	46.2
1962	360,250	130,000	404,000	40.3	14.5	45.2
1964	380,400	131,500	371,000	43.1	14.9	42.0
1966	409,720	164,100	513,000	37.7	15.1	47.2
1968	445,253	185,000	546,000	37.8	15.7	46.4
1970	472,000[d]	222,000	560,000	37.6	17.7	46.7
1972	499,594	270,000	597,000	36.6	20.0	43.7

[a]Sources, American Nurses Association, *Facts About Nursing*, various issues.
[b]Estimated. The figures on PNs and attendants were aggregated to 1952. In 1950, there were 181,647 PNs and attendants, 64,634 NAs, and 24,543 orderlies. From 1952–1956, PNs and attendants, NAs, and orderlies were shown separately, and from 1957–1959, NAs and attendants were aggregated. From 1960 on, attendants, orderlies, and NAs were all listed as NAs.
[c]Estimated extrapolation between 1956–1962. No figures on the numbers of PNs or NAs in hospitals are available for 1960 and 1961.
[d]Estimated, less nursing home workers.

of all RNs were female; in 1972, 98.6 per cent. About 97 per cent of PNs are women. It is only among NAs that there are a significant number of males, and this is largely because an important function of orderlies and attendants is to do heavier work such as lifting bodies and because a cheap male labor supply made up of blacks, chicanos, and Puerto Ricans has become available in urban areas since World War II (36).

The growing supplies of RNs and PNs actively employed are due not only to the expansion of RN and PN training programs, but also to the higher labor force participation rate of women in general and, in this case, nursing workers. (In 1957, the proportion of all women in the U.S. employed or actively seeking employment was 36.9 per cent; in 1974, 45.9 per cent (4).) That is, more of those who are trained to be nurses remain in the labor force for longer periods of time than previously. This is especially true of married women who now stay in the labor force longer both because of economic necessity and because of a desire to attain a wider social experience than is available as a houseworker.

In 1940, 46.4 per cent of all working women in the U.S. were married; in 1972, 63.3 per cent (4). Table 8 shows that the same trend has characterized the labor force participation status of the nursing labor force. Although the vast majority of RNs who are inactive are married, the proportion of RNs who are active has grown significantly since the late 1940s as has the percentage of active RNs who are married.

Table 8

The activity status and marital status of RNs,[a] 1949-1972[b]

Year	Active	Inactive	Per cent Active	Active Married	Active Divorced, Widowed, and Separated	Active Single	Inactive Married	Inactive Divorced, Widowed, and Separated	Inactive Single
	no.	no.	%	%	%	%	%	%	%
1949	300,533	205,517	59.3	41.9	10.3	46.4	87.0	3.4	8.3
1951	334,733	221,884	60.1	46.5	9.7	38.7	85.9	3.4	6.8
1957	464,138	231,834	66.7	55.2	9.8	31.4	86.2	4.6	5.9
1962	532,118	282,819	65.3	61.0	11.0	25.6	84.7	4.8	5.3
1966	593,694	285,791	67.5	63.5	11.5	22.4	86.4	5.8	5.7
1972	780,000	316,611	71.1	68.7	12.0	18.4	84.7	7.8	6.0

[a]Numbers of active and inactive nurses include some who did not report marital status. A 1927 survey of nursing schools showed that 20 per cent of their active graduates were married and 80 per cent unmarried in that year (13, p. 244). In 1943, an ANA tabulation showed that 65.8 per cent of RNs were active, of whom 39.6 per cent were listed as married and 60.4 per cent as unmarried (30, p. 8).
[b]Sources, reference 6; *Health Manpower Sourcebook*, Section 2, Nursing Personnel, p. 22. Department of Health, Education, and Welfare, January 1966.

Most active PNs are also married, although the percentage of those married does not appear to be as high as that for RNs. In a survey taken in 1967, 58.2 per cent of all employed PNs were married, 16.3 per cent were single, and 23.7 per cent were widowed, divorced, or separated (37). The high percentage of employed PNs in the latter category reflects the fact that many untrained women who are forced to enter the labor force later in life due to a change in marital status will often find the relatively short PN training period course the economically feasible alternative. PNs tend to be somewhat older than RNs, the mean age for the former in 1967 being about 43 years and that for the latter in 1966 being about 40 years (37; 38, p. 16).

The increasing tendency of RNs to stay in the nursing labor force is also reflected in the changes in the average age of nurses since the 1940s. Table 9 shows that, despite the rapid and steady growth in the number of RNs in the last 30 years (which in itself would tend to increase the proportions of nurses in the younger categories), the age distribution of active nurses has shifted sharply to older categories.

Table 9

Age distribution in per cent of active nurses, 1943–1972[a]

Age	1943	1949	1951	1957	1962	1966	1972
Total	100.0	100.0	100.0	100.0	100.0	100.0	100.0
Under 30	} 64.0	39.3	36.0	29.6	24.8	25.5	24.9
30–39		25.7	25.2	24.6	24.5	22.2	23.0
40–44	10.7	11.2	12.0	10.4	11.6	12.6	10.6
45–49		7.9	8.1	10.6	11.3	10.9	11.8
50–59	} 25.2	11.0	10.9	13.4	17.7	17.8	16.5
60 and over		3.6	4.1	6.6	7.1	7.9	8.8
Unknown		1.3	3.7	4.8	3.0	3.1	4.4

[a]Sources, references 6, Table I-A-8; 30, p. 8; 38, p. 21; *Health Manpower Sourcebook*, p. 20. Department of Health, Education, and Welfare, January 1966.

Table 10 demonstrates the activity status of RNs in terms of the changing ratios of active to inactive RNs in different age groups between 1949 and 1972. We see that for all age groups under 55, the ratio of active to inactive RNs has risen since 1949, with the extent of the increases being greatest in the younger age groups and least in the older age groups. We see a decline in the ratio for those over 60 since about 1957 (and an absolute decline compared to 1949), reflecting old-age benefits in the form of government welfare and industrial pension plans which were expanded in the 1960s. Among the under-60 groups, the lowest ratio is for those in the 30-39 age group. What

Table 10

Ratios of active to inactive RNs, 1949–1972[a]

Age Group	1949	1951	1957	1962	1966	1972
Under 25	–[b]	–	–	–	6.61	10.77
25–29	–	–	–	–	2.07	3.49
Under 30	1.73	1.74	2.79	2.33	2.94	4.45
30–34	–	–	–	–	1.37	1.93
35–39	–	–	–	–	1.52	1.97
30–39	0.98	1.04	1.32	1.33	1.44	1.95
40–44	1.47	1.51	1.90	1.82	1.95	2.45
45–49	2.02	1.95	2.19	2.51	2.54	2.84
50–54	–	–	–	–	2.87	2.87
55–59	–	–	–	–	2.87	2.57
50–59	2.32	2.28	2.74	2.76	2.87	2.73
60 and over	1.44	1.99	2.17	1.49	1.51	1.25

[a]Sources, references 6, Table I-A-8; 30, p. 8; 38, p. 21; *Health Manpower Sourcebook*, p. 20. Department of Health, Education, and Welfare, January 1966.
[b]Dash signifies data not available before 1966.

this table indicates is that many RNs still drop out of the labor force to have children but then reenter the labor force when their children start going to school.

With this increased labor force participation, RNs are more likely to see their employment conditions (i.e. the level of wages, work relations, and the quality of patient care) in a longer-run perspective than previously. Moreover, women who are permanently in the labor force will tend to have a different consciousness of male-female relations than women who fluctuate between the family home and the nursing workplace (especially those who do not do so out of economic necessity), or than women who see the nursing workplace as simply a way station on the route to a family home. The permanent wage-workers are more likely to reject the traditional ideology of female submissiveness to males which has been very functional for maintaining and manipulating the hierarchical order of the health industry. Hence, with increased labor force participation on the part of RNs, and the nursing labor force in general, important *objective conditions* have come into being for the organization of these workers to change their work conditions, and the quality of health care delivery. A better basis exists for the raising of feminist and socialist consciousness among nursing workers and the building of action-oriented workers' organizations.

Racial Divisions in the Nursing Hierarchy

The hierarchical structure of authority in the health industry is most marked in terms of the control which men (doctors) exercise over women (nurses). However, in the U.S. the hierarchical division of labor also exists along racial lines *within* the nursing labor force; i.e. RNs (who give orders to PNs and NAs) are still dispropor-tionately white (relative to the number of blacks, chicanos, Puerto Ricans, and American Indians in the U.S. labor force in general). In 1950, only 3.5 per cent of female RNs were non-white. As we have seen, in the 1940s the hospitals began to recognize the potential for filling NA positions with the large number of blacks who were coming out of the rural areas into the cities.

Today blacks are much more integrated into the lower levels of the nursing labor force hierarchy. In fact they are disproportionately represented (relative to their numbers in the labor force) at the PN and NA levels. In 1970, black women constituted about 12 per cent of the experienced female labor force, but over 25 per cent of all female NAs and about 22 per cent of all female PNs. They were underrepresented among RNs, constituting 7.3 per cent of all female RNs (which, however, was more than double the percentage in 1950) (39).

This integration of blacks into the RN labor force will probably go further in the future (although the number of blacks will still remain relatively larger at the lower levels of the nursing labor force in general). As nursing education has shifted more and more out of the hospital setting and into the public system of higher education, it has become more accessible to blacks. Table 11 shows that a much larger proportion of students entering and graduating from A.D. and B.S. programs in recent years have been blacks.

As blacks become more integrated into the RN nursing work force, it will be much more difficult for employers to use racist ideology to keep different groups of workers apart. When hierarchical divisions such as those between RNs, PNs, and NAs are also black-white divisions, notions of white superiority tend to reinforce notions of

Table 11

Black as a percentage of all students entering and graduating from initial
nursing programs in the United States, 1962–1972[a]

Year	Practical E[b]	G[c]	A.D. E	G	Diploma E	G	B.S. E	G	All Initial RN Programs E	G
1962–1963	16.4	12.0	5.2	5.6	2.4	2.3	4.9	9.7	3.0	3.4
1965–1966	18.1	16.3	6.5	6.1	2.0	2.4	4.8	4.0	3.2	3.0
1968–1969	17.4	15.5	10.5	6.0	3.6	2.0	6.0	4.0	6.2	3.2
1971–1972	16.8	15.8	10.9	10.1	4.1	3.3	10.3	5.0	8.5	6.3

[a]Sources, Educational preparation for nursing–1969. *Nursing Outlook* 18-19: 56, September 1970.
reference 6, p. 88.

[b]E–Entering.
[c]G–Graduating.

occupational superiority. As the black-white divisions break down, the legitimacy of
such racist notions is more easily questioned and rejected.

Social Concentration of Nursing Workers

Along with the greater labor force participation of RNs and the integration of
blacks into the RN nursing labor force, the increasing concentration of nursing workers
in large-scale work settings has also created more favorable objective conditions for
worker organization and action. Tables 12 through 14 show the changes in the
percentage distribution of RNs from 1949 to 1972 and of PNs and NAs from 1962 to
1972 in various types of work settings.

Table 12

Percentage distribution of registered nurses by type of work, 1949–1972[a]

Type of Work	1949	1951	1956–58	1962	1964	1966	1968	1970	1972
Hospital	{48.5	{50.0	{59.8	65.5	65.3	66.0	66.8	65.4	65.2
Nursing home				1.3	1.7	1.8	2.7	6.5	7.0
Nursing school	2.6	2.3	2.4	3.5	3.5	3.7	3.7	3.5	3.8
Public health[b]	9.7	8.9	7.1	6.3	6.4	6.5	7.1	7.1	9.0
Occupational health[c]	4.4	4.3	3.8	3.1	3.2	2.9	2.9	2.8	2.5
Private duty[d]	21.6	20.9	15.0	12.6	11.3				
Office	8.8	8.4	8.0	7.3	8.1	}19.2	}16.8	}14.7	}12.5
Other and unclassified	3.9	5.2	3.9	0.4	0.3				

[a]Source, American Nurses Association, *Facts About Nursing*, various issues.
[b]Workplaces are usually in public institutions such as schools and clinics.
[c]Workplaces are in industrial settings.
[d]Workplaces are in private homes and in hospitals and nursing homes (private bedside care).

With the continued shift of health care delivery from the home to the hospital, the
percentage of RNs in nonbureaucratic workplaces (homes, small offices) has declined
dramatically (from well over 30 per cent in 1949 to about 13 per cent in 1972). Also,
the shift of PNs to the hospital and nursing home settings which began in the 1940s

Table 13

Percentage distribution of practical nurses by type of work, 1962–1972[a]

Type of Work	1962	1964	1966	1968	1970	1972
Hospital	{ 57.8	52.6	58.2	57.8	60.0	63.2
Nursing home		8.2	12.1	14.1	14.9	17.1
Public health[b]	0.2	0.2	0.3	0.6	0.8	0.9
Private duty,[c] office, and other	42.0	39.0	29.4	27.6	24.4	18.7

[a]Source, reference 6, Table IV-A-7.
[b]Workplaces are usually in public institutions such as schools and clinics.
[c]Workplaces are in private homes and in hospitals and nursing homes (private bedside care).

Table 14

Percentage distribution of nursing aides by type of work, 1962–1972[a]

Type of Work	1962	1964	1966	1968	1970	1972
Hospital	{ 98.5	74.2	73.3	70.5	67.5	66.3
Nursing home		24.2	25.3	27.7	30.5	31.1
Public health[b]	1.0	1.2	1.1	1.5	1.8	2.3
Other	0.5	0.4	0.3	0.3	0.2	0.2

[a]Source, reference 6, Table IV-B-1.
[b]Home health aides.

and 1950s has continued steadily to the present. NAs (including orderlies and attendants) who had traditionally worked in nursing homes, and whose labor was developed in the 1940s specifically for hospitals, remain firmly entrenched in these workplaces.

The rapid expansion of both the number and proportion of RNs, PNs, and NAs in nursing homes in the late 1960s is largely due to the introduction of Medicare and Medicaid. In 1972, 7.9 per cent of all RNs listed geriatric nursing as their area of clinical practice (6, Table I-7-A). Between 1963 and 1971, the number of nursing care and related homes in the U.S. increased by 35 per cent (from 16,701 to 22,588), while the number of beds increased by 117 per cent (from an average of 34 beds per home to 55 beds per home). Most of this increase was due to the establishment of proprietary nursing homes, which comprised 78 per cent of all nursing homes and held 67 per cent of all nursing beds in 1971 (5, pp. 385-396).

Educational Credentials of Nursing Workers

As we have discussed above, the movement of nursing workers into more impersonal, concentrated, and profit-oriented workplaces has been accompanied by attempts on the part of health employers to establish hierarchical divisions of labor which create an optimal balance between competition and cooperation among workers: competition keeping workers *divided politically*, and cooperation keeping workers *united technically*. As part of this process, educational credentials have assumed utmost importance in channeling people into different levels of the hierarchy and in legitimizing the resulting lines of authority and allocation of job functions (40, 41).

The ANA has, since the Goldmark Report, held to the principle that PNs should be trained, but that their training should be kept separate and quite distinct from RN training (22, p. 28). Over the last decade or so, however, both PN training and lower-level RN training have been moving increasingly into the community colleges (see Tables 15 through 17). Although the PN and RN programs remain distinct, the possibility is increased that those RNs with associate degrees might find themselves with educational credentials little distinguishable from those held by community college-trained PNs. As it is, their actual functions overlap to a great extent.

Table 15

Distribution of initial registered nurses' programs by institutional control, 1955–1972[a]

Year	All Schools		University and College		Hospital		Junior or Community College		Independent	
	no.	%	no.	%	no.	%	no.	%	no.	%
1955	1139	100.0	180	15.8	959[b]	84.2				
1961	1118	100.0	245	21.9	873[b]	78.1				
1968	1287	100.0	301	23.4	696	54.1	251	19.5	39	3.0
1971	1350	100.0	395	29.3	565	41.9	364	27.0	26	1.9
1972	1363	100.0	409	30.0	524	38.4	408	29.9	22	1.6

[a]Source, American Nurses Association, *Facts About Nursing*, various issues.
[b]Includes a small number of community colleges and independent schools.

Table 16

Distribution of practical nurses' programs by administrative control, 1960-1972[a]

Year	All Schools		Technical, Trade, and Vocational		University, College, and Junior College		Hospital		Secondary		Other		Total Enrollments
	no.	%	no.	%	no.	%	no.	%	no.	%	no.	%	no.
1960	693	100.0	438	63.2	52	7.5	190	27.4	0	0.0	13	1.9	23,817
1967	1149	100.0	624	54.3	188	16.4	234	20.4	76	6.6	27	2.3	44,292
1971	1291	100.0	682	52.8	275	21.3	194	15.0	89	6.9	51	4.0	58,186
1972	1310	100.0	690	52.7	304	23.2	176	13.4	89	6.8	51	3.9	n.a.[b]

[a]Sources, reference 6, Table IV-C-3; reference 38, p. 170; American Nurses Association, *Facts About Nursing*, 1962–1963, p. 183, 1969, p. 170, 1972–1973, Table IV-C-3.
[b]n.a. signifies data not available.

Since the great expansion of hospital RNs in the 1940s, the hospital employers and the nursing elite (administrators and some educators) have been trying to draw the distinction between the "professional" RN (who has at least a college degree) and the "technical" (rank-and-file) RN (33, p. 92; 42). The movement to downgrade (in terms of control over work and relative pay) the RN with the A.D. is facilitated as the number of RNs with B.S. degrees expands. In 1954, 24,215 students, or 21.2 per cent of all students in RN training programs, were enrolled in B.S. nursing programs. In 1972, over 83,160 students, or 36.3 per cent of all nursing students, were enrolled in these programs. Not all or even the major proportion of B.S. graduates can become teachers, administrators, or supervisors (as was previously the case). Some will occupy

Table 17

Percentage distribution of students enrolled at various levels of
registered nurses' education, 1950–1972[a]

Year	A.D.	Diploma	B.S. Initial	B.S. (2nd Degree)	Master's	Doctorate	Total No. Enrolled
1950	[b]	81.1	7.7	11.2[c]			110,284
1954	[d]	77.4	12.8	8.4	1.4[e]		114,226
1958	1.5	73.2	15.2	8.1	2.0	0.1	126,338
1962	3.6	70.4	17.5	6.6	1.8	0.1	135,409
1964	6.0	65.7	19.5	6.6	2.0	0.1	141,637
1966	10.2	60.1	21.9	5.4	2.3	0.1	150,933
1968	17.4	49.3	25.6	5.0	2.5	0.2	157,713
1970	25.1	40.1	27.6	4.3	2.7	0.2	177,314
1971	28.0	35.6	29.8	3.8	2.7	0.1	200,949
1972	29.5	31.3	32.3	4.0	2.8	0.2	229,094

[a]Sources, reference 6, Tables II-A-14, II-C-1; reference 32, pp. 75, 95, 98; reference 38, pp. 90, 109.
[b]Introduced in 1952.
[c]Includes enrollments in Master's and Doctoral programs.
[d]Less than 1 per cent of diploma total. In 1955, A.D. students were 1.1 per cent of all diploma students.
[e]Includes enrollments in Doctoral programs.

(or move up to) these roles, but with further "inflation" of educational credentials, those with master's and doctoral degrees will have an ever-tighter monopoly on these positions. For the present, the B.S. RNs will be used at the staff nurse level to downgrade the A.D. RNs. But with the creation of further divisions in the nursing work force, B.S. RNs themselves will be vulnerable to downgrading as their numbers expand.

The increase in the number of both B.S. graduates and A.D. graduates reflects the decline of the hospital school with its intermediate three-year program. With the expansion of full-time nursing workers in hospitals, and with the growing specialization of functions, the use of student nurses as a source of labor has become increasingly unimportant to hospitals. At the same time, the hospital schools have become dispensable in the training of the RN labor supply as the U.S. system of higher education, and especially the community college track of that system (43), has expanded since World War II. Hospitals no longer have the incentive or the need to bear the expenses of training RNs, and the hospital-based diploma program is slowly being phased out (44, Ch. IV). In 1970–1971, 54 diploma programs were terminated and there were no new additions, and 80 programs were in the process of closing down (42). Between 1968 and 1972, the number of hospital schools decreased by almost 25 per cent (see Table 15).

There were other reasons for the shift to colleges and community colleges, notably the attitudes of potential students toward the diploma programs. Many students prefer the B.S. programs to diploma programs because a B.S. degree provides flexibility to the graduate nurse in terms of mobility both within and outside the occupation of nursing. Other students who cannot qualify for B.S. programs or who cannot afford to go to college for 4 years often prefer the A.D. program because it is shorter and because it does not require that they take up residence in a hospital.

Further Development of the Nursing Labor Force

In the first section of this article, we presented a quantitative picture of the general hierarchical structure in the "average" hospital. In Table 18 we demonstrate the quantitative development of the hierarchical structure since 1946. It will be seen that the number of people in all positions in the actual delivery of patient care has increased markedly, while the number of instructors has declined sharply and the number of administrators has risen only slightly. Significant, once again, are the sharp increase in the number of PNs and the less dramatic increase in the number of NAs in the average hospital. It should also be noted that the number of RNs at the staff nurse level in the average hospital fell between 1970 and 1972, while this decline was more than compensated by the increase in the numbers of PNs and NAs. Here we have a broad indication of the substitution of "low-priced" labor for "high-priced" labor.

Table 18

Hierarchical structure of the nursing labor force in hospitals, 1946-1972[a,b]

Category	1946	1950	1954	1958	1962	1966	1970	1972
Administration								
Directors and assistants	1.34	1.51	1.66	1.96	1.62	1.52	1.78	1.91
Other administrative personnel					0.42	0.28	0.22	0.28
Instructors	0.66	0.86	1.17	1.54	2.05	3.14	2.45	0.96
Patient care								
Supervisors and assistants	2.91	3.40	3.84	4.51	4.62	3.97	4.64	7.29
Head nurses and assistants	4.07	5.04	6.36	7.32	8.04	8.39	9.35	12.23
Staff nurses	12.44	18.42	22.79	24.61	27.01	29.21	37.12	35.54
Practical nurses			10.00	13.23	17.58	20.85	28.75	35.18
Nursing aides, orderlies, attendants	21.23	36.52	43.49	43.51	55.93	67.47	73.58	79.48

[a]Source, American Nurses Association, *Facts About Nursing,* various issues.
[b]For 1946, 1950, and 1954, only staff nurses are calculated in full-time equivalents. For 1958, 1962, 1966, 1970, and 1972, all levels are calculated in full-time equivalents.

Over the past 25 years, rearrangements of job structures have characterized the health industry, as, in accordance with the "Ginzberg" principle cited earlier, various functions have been shifted to cheaper labor (9, Ch. 12; 29; 31; 35; 45; 46). What this principle tells employers is to cut labor costs wherever possible. Underlying this seemingly simple dictum is the whole basis for conflict between employers and employees, and at times between different strata of employees, not only in the health industry, but in any industry which is run along capitalistic lines. First, it is assumed that the decision making involved in work reorganization is made at the top of the hierarchy; that is, employers make decisions and give orders, employees carry them out. Second, the definition of "low-priced work" is an outcome of this authoritarian decision-making process. "Low-priced work" has no separate existence (except, perhaps, in the minds of employers) from "low-priced labor"; and in reality such work only becomes so defined when there is cheap labor available to do the work. If it is not available, employers understand that it has to be *made available,* or alternatively replaced by cost-cutting machines (where this is possible), if they want to get the same work done at less cost.

Organizing for Better Health Care

The service character of the health industry makes it difficult to carry mechanization of health care delivery too far, although ultimately it is the organized efforts of health workers and the consumers of health care, and not technology, which block the introduction of mechanization which threatens to further depersonalize the delivery of health services. The substitution of lower-priced supplies of labor (i.e. labor which is relatively abundant and which has little bargaining power) for higher-priced supplies of labor is therefore the primary mode of achieving "cost-efficient" operations in the health industry.

The extent to which plans for cost-reducing (and profit-making) rearrangements of the division of labor in the health industry can go forward depends on the opposition to or the support for these plans on the part of health workers on the one hand, and the consumers of health care on the other.

The health industry is more profitable now than ever, the cost of health care to consumers is continually rising, and the quality of health services is severely deficient. When "cost-efficient" methods of work reorganization result in lower quality and/or quantity of health care services, the consumers of these services have little power. As *consumers,* they are isolated from one another (since in capitalist society, consumption is done in a highly individualized framework). They are also deprived of medical knowledge, and are consequently either susceptible to the mystique of the medical powers of doctors, or, with experience, just cynical about the possibilities of attaining good health care.

With the economy in recession, making health insurance premiums and other health costs an excessive burden on more and more people, the cost and quality of health care has become an ever more important political issue at both the national and industrial levels. Under such conditions, effective consumer action groups may emerge. However, on the demand side of health care, it will be organizations of *workers* rather than organizations of *consumers* which will wield more power in a movement for better and less expensive health care. As labor unions demand health coverage for their workers and as large industries and institutions set up Health Maintenance Organizations, the costs of health care services are increasingly being recognized as an *essential* part of the subsistence expenditure of workers, required for the reproduction of their labor, rather than as a type of discretionary spending of these workers as "consumers."

Organizing for Better Working Conditions

The pressure of consumer groups and worker organizations outside the health industry is vital to any movement to restructure the health care delivery system. But progressive and enduring changes require that the workers on the supply side of health care, i.e. those who do the actual work of delivering health care, develop a unity among themselves which will permit them to challenge the power of health employers and unite with other worker and consumer groups in a movement for change. Here the nursing work force is in a *potentially* powerful position. (So are doctors. It is our view, however, that while many doctors are supporting, and more will support, movements for decent health care, doctors as a group benefit too much from the present system, and are too socialized into it, to be counted on to play a major role in a movement to change it.) But the effective use of that power is seriously undermined by the hierarchical divisions between RNs and PNs, and among RNs themselves. These divisions were illustrated in a relatively militant strike of 4400 RNs in 41 San Francisco hospitals and clinics in June 1974 (47). Besides the usual wage demands, a primary demand in this strike was for more RN control over the work process. PNs, NAs, and other lower-level hospital workers felt uneasy about supporting the strike because they saw RNs as trying to strengthen, rather than break down, the existing hierarchical division of labor. On the other hand, RNs, as a result of their professional image of themselves, were uneasy about *accepting* the support of these workers because they did not want to commit themselves to supporting any similar actions which PNs, NAs, and others might take in the future.

The Need for Unity

Such divisions in the nursing work force must be overcome if these health workers are to exert some control over the quality of health care and over the nature of their own jobs. A movement for better health services and a movement for more worker control over the health industry are parts of the same struggle. Among nursing workers, RNs, by virtue of their increasing role in the delivery of health services previously in the domain of medical practice (e.g. the recent development of the pediatric nurse[1] and the nurse-midwife[2]), are in a key position to organize this struggle and carry it forward. Although they do not at present have the power to make *essential* decisions related to work organization and health care delivery (such as the quality and quantity of workers to be employed, who will be hired and who will be fired, the quality and quantity of health care that will be delivered, the establishment of lines of authority, the allocation of jobs), they do occupy positions of responsibility and authority both over other workers and over the actual day-to-day delivery of health care within the hierarchical order. At present, the use of this responsibility and authority serves the interests of RNs to some extent and the interests of health employers to an even greater extent. What is required is the development of worker

[1] Many doctors have found that they could profitably extend "their" practices by shifting the day-to-day work of immunizations and examinations of children onto RNs, while large health institutions have been able to dispense with doctors and use cheaper nurse labor for these functions (48, 49). The profit potential of using these nurses is most vivid in private medical practices where the net contribution of a nurse to profits can be easily separated out. For example, in one private practice, the addition of a pediatric nurse at a cost of $7,620 (she was paid about 40 per cent more than other RNs in the office) permitted an increase in patient visits by 18.8 per cent and brought in $16,800, for an annual net profit of over $9,000 (49).

[2] Midwives, although outlawed in many states in the first decades of this century, have continued to exist in thinly populated and very poor areas. Their numbers, however, have been steadily decreasing. In 1935, 10.7 per cent of all births were attended by midwives; in 1968, 1.0 per cent (5, p. 9). In 1948 there were 20,700 midwives in the U.S.; in 1971, 3,552 (of which 96 per cent were in the South, and almost 63 per cent in Texas, Arkansas, and Alabama alone) (5, pp. 210-211). Recently, however, doctors and hospitals have started to give this function back to women, not as independent practitioners as were the midwives, but as employees of doctors and health institutions (5, p. 209). In 1971, there were about 1,250 *nurse-midwives* in the U.S. with about 85 annual graduates from the nine schools which offered programs.

organizations which will provide a structure for RNs to utilize this authority and responsibility in the service of all health workers and health consumers.

Most health workers, including RNs, are not organized into unions, although some headway has been made in the last few years. In 1974, less than 300,000 out of 1.5 million health workers in 3,300 nonprofit, private hospitals belonged to unions (50). (There were several unions organizing these workers. While this sometimes permits workers to choose between unions, the inter-union rivalry that results leads to a great weakening of the labor movement.) RNs, insofar as they have collective bargaining agents, are usually represented by their State Nurses Associations. (In 1970, just 8.1 per cent of RNs, or 38,116, were covered by contracts negotiated by these Associations) (44, p. 15).) As was demonstrated by the San Francisco strike, these Associations, representing as they do only the RNs, weaken nursing workers in general by dividing them further. What is required if workers are to exert a significant measure of control over the work processes and output of the health industry are worker organizations which will allow all the wage-workers in the health sector to sort out the problems between them *before* they confront their employers rather than *while* certain groups of workers are confronting their employers. Such a united front will require that RNs, or at least the vast majority of rank-and-file RNs who do not occupy positions in the upper levels of the nursing hierarchy, reject the false ideology of professionalism and recognize the character of their own alienated work conditions.

Tendencies and Possibilities

How the development of such worker organizations can be carried forward must rely on much closer analyses which take into account the specific circumstances of each work situation. What we have demonstrated on a general level is that the changing objective conditions facing the nursing labor force present many favorable opportunities for such organization. Over the past century, the nursing labor force has developed from a relatively small number of isolated individuals working mostly in private homes to over 2 million workers concentrated together in large, hierarchically structured enterprises. The changing structure of the nursing labor force and the changing social relations of nursing work are consistent with, and part of the process of, the much larger development of the capitalist system in the U.S. into its monopolistic stage. In recent years, the structure of monopoly capitalism has begun to weaken seriously (the analysis of which is beyond the scope of this paper). Just as during the depression of the 1930s, industrial workers in the U.S. saw the necessity of taking militant action to gain basic rights of labor organization and bargaining, so too in the current period of recession and inflation will workers in key service industries such as health find the idea of united action more and more compelling in the face of eroding standards of living. How effective such action is will depend in large measure on the organizational forms which it takes and on the unity of purpose which is achieved and sustained.

We have argued in the preceding pages that the objective conditions for worker organization in the health industry have become more favorable over the last decade. Health workers, and primarily nursing workers, are playing an ever-increasing role in the actual delivery of health care, both absolutely and relative to doctors. At the same time, they are increasingly concentrated in large institutional work units, making mass organization against a common employer, or a relatively small number of employers, possible. Further, nursing workers are staying in the labor force longer, and hence have a stronger commitment to changing the conditions of their work. Meanwhile, it appears that racial divisions in the nursing labor force, which have been useful to employers in setting one group of workers against another, have been breaking down at the rank-and-file nursing levels over the last decade. In addition, the structure of educational credentials, which is utilized to channel workers into different levels of the nursing hierarchy and to legitimize the hierarchical division of labor, is corresponding less and less to the actual structure of work relations among rank-and-file nurses. Finally, increasing numbers of nursing workers are being concentrated at the lower levels of the nursing hierarchy.

It must be emphasized that these changing objective conditions are tendencies which we perceive in the development of the nursing labor force and that we have analyzed these conditions at a very aggregated level. A clearer understanding of how these tendencies will develop requires a more in-depth and more disaggregated analysis. What we have presented here is intended as a general framework for such an analysis. It must also be emphasized that the importance of these objective conditions for the development of worker organizations and for a radical restructuring of the system of health care delivery can only be assessed in conjunction with an analysis of the subjective forces which are necessary to transform possibilities into practice. The women's movement and the feminist consciousness which it engenders are valuable in helping to forge the unity necessary to take advantage of the objective conditions facing the nursing labor force. But if any steps forward are to be of lasting significance, this consciousness itself must be developed into a socialist perspective on the delivery of health care and its relation to the rest of the capitalist system.

Acknowledgments—We would like to thank Sam Baker, Howard Berliner, Carol Brown, Barbara Caress, Joel Denker, Grace Kleinbach, Helen Marieskind, and Susan Reverby for their helpful criticism and advice.

REFERENCES

1. Bodenheimer, T., Cummings, S., and Harding, E., editors. *Billions for Band-Aids*. Medical Committee for Human Rights, San Francisco, 1972.
2. Waitzkin, H., and Waterman, B. *The Exploitation of Illness in Capitalist Society*. Bobbs-Merrill, Indianapolis, 1974.
3. Ehrenreich, B., and Ehrenreich, J. *The American Health Empire: Power, Profits, and Politics*. Vintage, New York, 1971.
4. Economic Affairs Bureau. *Dollars & Sense* No. 2, pp. 6-7, 13, December 1974.
5. U.S. Department of Health, Education, and Welfare, Public Health Service. *Health Resources Statistics; Health Manpower and Health Facilities, 1972-1973*. U.S. Government Printing Office, Washington, D. C., 1973.
6. *Facts About Nursing, 1972-1973*. American Nurses Association, New York, 1973.
7. Edwards, R. C. Bureaucratic organization in the capitalist firm. In *The Capitalist System*, edited by R. Edwards, M. Reich, and T. Weisskopf, pp. 115-119. Prentice-Hall, Englewood Cliffs, N.J., 1972.
8. *Health Occupations Supportive to Nursing*, p. 6. American Nurses Association, New York, 1965.
9. Alexander, E. L. *Nursing Administration in the Hospital Health Care System*. C. V. Mosby, St. Louis, 1972.
10. U.S. Department of Labor. *Dictionary of Occupational Titles*, pp. 493-494. U.S. Government Printing Office, Washington, D. C., 1965.

11. Salaries in community health services, 1972. *Nursing Outlook,* p. 20, December 1972.
12. Silver, G. Caspar Weinberger's bitter pill. *The Nation,* pp. 276-277, September 24, 1973.
13. Burgess, M. A. *Nurses, Patients, and Pocketbooks.* Committee on the Grading of Nursing Schools, New York, 1928.
14. U.S. Bureau of the Census. *Historical Statistics of the United States From Colonial Times to 1957.* U.S. Government Printing Office, Washington, D. C., 1959.
15. Shryock, R. *The History of Nursing,* pp. 219, 288-305. Saunders, Philadelphia, 1959.
16. Jamieson, E., and Sewall, M. *Trends in Nursing History,* Ed. 3, p. 303. Saunders, Washington, D. C., 1949.
17. English, D., and Ehrenreich, B. *Witches, Midwives and Nurses: A History of Women Healers,* pp. 21-34. Glass Mountain, Oyster Bay, N.Y, 1972.
18. Jensen, D. *History and Trends of Professional Nursing,* Ed. 4. Mosby, St. Louis, 1959.
19. Strachey, R. *Struggle: The Stirring Story of Woman's Advance in England,* pp. 23-29, 46, 71. Duffield, New York, 1930.
20. Bullough, V., and Bullough, B. *The Emergence of Modern Nursing,* Ed. 2. Macmillan, New York, 1969.
21. Dock, L. The relation of training schools to hospitals. In *Hospitals, Dispensaries, and Nursing,* pp. 86-96, International Congress of Charities, Correction and Philanthropy, Johns Hopkins Press, Baltimore, 1894.
22. Committee for the Study of Nursing Education (Goldmark Report). *Nursing and Nursing Education in the United States.* Macmillan, New York, 1923.
23. Ashley, J.A. This I believe about power in nursing. *Nursing Outlook* 21(10): 637-641, 1973.
24. Deming, D. *The Practical Nurse.* Commonwealth Fund, New York, 1943.
25. Stewart, I. *The Education of Nurses.* Macmillan, New York, 1943.
26. Flexner, A. *Medical Education in the United States and Canada,* pp. 151-152. Updike, Boston, 1910.
27. Stevens, R. *American Medicine and the Public Interest,* pp. 54-74. Yale University Press, New Haven, 1971.
28. Markowitz, G., and Rosner, D. Doctors in crisis: A study of the use of medical education reform to establish modern professional elitism in medicine. *American Quarterly* 25: 83-107, March 1973.
29. Baker, E. *Technology and Woman's Work,* pp. 312, 321. Columbia University Press, New York, 1964.
30. *Facts About Nursing, 1943.* American Nurses Association, New York, 1943.
31. Brown, C. The division of laborers: Allied health professions. *Int. J. Health Serv.* 3(3): 435-444, 1973.
32. *Facts About Nursing, 1955-56,* pp. 162-163. American Nurses Association, New York, 1956.
33. Brown, E. L. *Nursing for the Future,* pp. 66-67. Russell Sage Foundation, New York, 1948.
34. Hughes, E., Hughes, H., and Deutscher, I. *Twenty Thousand Nurses Tell Their Story.* Lippincott, Philadelphia, 1958.
35. Reverby, S. Health: Women's work. *Health/PAC Bulletin* 40: 15-20, April 1972.
36. Ehrenreich, J., and Ehrenreich, B. Hospital workers: A case study in the "new working class." *Monthly Review* 24(8): 12-27, 1973.
37. Marshall, E., and Moses, E. *An Inventory of Licensed Practical Nurses—1967,* p. 33. U.S. Government Printing Office, Washington, D. C., 1971.
38. *Facts About Nursing, 1969.* American Nurses Association, New York, 1969.
39. U.S. Bureau of the Census. *1970 Census of the Population: Detailed Characteristics.* U.S. Government Printing Office, Washington, D. C., 1971.
40. Bowles, S. The integration of higher education into the wage labor system. *Review of Radical Political Economics* 6(1): 100-133, 1974.
41. Bowles, S., and Gintis, H. IQ in the U.S. class structure. *Social Policy* III(4 and 5): 65-96, January/February 1973.
42. Bayer, A. The quality promise of nursing education policy. *Educational Record* pp. 288-293, Fall 1973.
43. Karabel, J. Community colleges and social stratification. *Harvard Educational Review* 42(4): 521-562, 1972.
44. Altman, S. *Present and Future Supply of Registered Nurses.* U.S. Government Printing Office, Washington, D. C., 1971.
45. Beyers, M., and Phillips, C. *Nursing Management for Patient Care,* Ch. 8. Little, Brown, Boston, 1971.

46. U.S. Department of Health, Education, and Welfare. *Nursing Manpower Programs,* Ch. IV. 1968.
47. Gaynor, D., Blake, E., Bodenheimer, T., and Mermey, C. RN's strike. *Health/PAC Bulletin* 60: 1-6, 10-14, September/October 1974.
48. Andrews, P., and Yankauer, A. The pediatric nurse practitioner. *American Journal of Nursing* 71(3), March 1971.
49. Sadler, A., Sadler, B., and Bliss, A. *The Physician's Assistant,* pp. 35-37. Yale University Press, New Haven, 1972.
50. *Wall Street Journal,* p. 22, July 29, 1974.

CHAPTER 11

Women Workers In
The Health Service Industry
Carol A. Brown

Health work is women's work. Over 85 per cent of all health service and hospital workers are women. The largest occupation in health work—nursing—is almost entirely female.

The increase in health employment over the past decades has been primarily an increase in women employees. Weiss(1) showed that the occupations that were predominantly female were expanding fastest, and that most occupations were becoming increasingly female. He showed the reason to be that the greatest increase has been at the lower ends of the ladder, where there are more women. Between 1960 and 1970 the number of physicians in practice increased by only 25 per cent, registered nurses by 39 per cent, and practical nurses by 80 per cent(2).

The health service industry is run by a small minority. It is run primarily by physicians, who have traditionally held the power, but also by the increasingly powerful hospital administrators, insurance company directors, government regulators, medical school educators, and corporation managers. Most of these people are men(3).

Aside from this top level in which industrial power is concentrated, men are found largely at the bottom—as kitchen helpers, janitors, and porters—and in a few technical fields such as laboratory and x-ray. Men at the bottom experience the same lack of power as their female coworkers, and, like the women, the further down the professional ladder they are the more likely they are to be non-white.

Health service is women's work, but not women's power. It is not unusual to find industrial power concentrated at the top echelon of an industry, nor to find the policy or practice of "men only" at the top echelon. It *is* unusual to find an industry requiring a complex mix of highly technical skills in which most of the skilled as well as the unskilled workers are women. In health service the conflict between "management" and "workers" is a conflict mainly between men and women.

Three main areas are dealt with in this paper. First, why are health workers women? Second, how is the overlap of sexual and occupational status upheld, and with what effects on the field? Third, what struggles take place that may lead to change in the future?

THE EMPLOYMENT OF WOMEN

Many apparent advantages to physicians and other elites in the health industry accrue to the hiring of women. First, women are an inexpensive source of labor. Health care is a costly but essential commodity, with labor constituting the biggest expense. Health service only became big business with the rise of hospitals. Hospital services are expensive and the biggest expense is labor. If costs are beyond the reach of consumers, the industry suffers, and with it the incomes of physicians and service organizations. Public financing has been put forth as one solution to high health costs; keeping labor costs low is another. A labor force composed mostly of women can be hired more cheaply than one composed mostly of men. Women can be paid less than men would be paid for the same work. In addition, women are believed to be dedicated to service and not self-interest (4), and are expected to drop out of the labor force to raise families—thus obviating the need for promotions or increased pay for seniority (5).

Second, women are available. Rapid expansion of labor requires an easily available labor force to draw on, and women are the last major reservoir of unemployment (6).

Third, women are safe. They pose no threat to physicians who, in order to expand their own services and therefore their incomes, must be assured of subordinates who will stay subordinate. Women do not have the social power—that is, access to capital, access to specialized education, freedom from family responsibilities, and respect of political leaders—to become organized competition to physicians in the medical marketplace, whereas other men and other male-dominated professions such as optometry or osteopathy do provide competition to physicians (7). Women's efforts to open medical schools to more women students have had limited success for the same reasons. At an interpersonal level, physicians are (or hope to be) assured of respect and willing service in members of subordinate occupations in part because they are men and the others are women.

Why do women accept the low pay and interpersonal subordination of the health service industry? If asked, many would say they went into health service to help people, to care for the sick, rather than to earn a high salary or to enjoy prestige. Caring for others is seen as women's work by society at large, and is seen by many women as their vocation. But physicians and surgeons also help the sick. The answer to women's acceptance of poorly paid subordinate occupations lies outside the health service industry in the economic opportunities available to women elsewhere. Women are "willing" to accept subordinate conditions of work because they have little choice in the matter.

Few occupations are open to women, whereas many are open to men. Out of 80 major occupational categories listed in the 1970 United States Census, seven occupations contain 43 per cent of all women workers. One of these occupations is nursing (8). Non-white women are concentrated in service and labor occupations. Discrimination is endemic, and few can afford to spend years pressing anti-discrimination suits at every barrier. When people need jobs they have to take what is open to them. When they need skill training, they learn what skills are offered. In addition, most women work because they need the money. The majority of women workers are single, are sole supports of households, or have husbands with incomes below $4000 a year (9).

The low pay for high skills found in health service is only low compared to white *men's* opportunities elsewhere. From the point of view of women, the pay is relatively good. Pay rates are low in all occupations in all industries for women. Median full-time earnings in hospital employment are *above* the median for workers in all industries for the categories of white women, black men, and black women. Median earnings in hospital employment are well below the median only for white men (10). One black woman from the South described to this author her entry into health service as a nurses' aide as an "incredible opportunity," because it was steady work and good wages. In getting further education, the average woman does not have a choice between nursing school and medical school, but between nursing school and, for example, computer programming school.

The lack of promotion opportunities in health careers over a lifetime does not compare unfavorably to the lack of promotion opportunities everywhere else for women. Of all the managers and non-farm administrators at all levels in the economy, only 16 per cent are women and 1 per cent non-white women (11).

Women's low wages compared to men's make a wife-mother necessarily dependent on her husband for her livelihood and that of her children (12). Her husband has the economic power to insist that she give up any other job. Thus, because of her tenuous position, long-term upward mobility opportunities within one organization, as much as she might want them, become unavailable to her. More relevant are good starting pay and certified skills for jobs that she can leave, reenter, and move to a new location. In many health occupations, one-half of entrants have left after five years; those who remain often change jobs for marginally higher pay, better working conditions, or family responsibilities, rather than for nonexistent promotion opportunities (13, 14).

Women accept the interpersonal subordination assigned to them in health service for the same reasons they accept low pay: there is a lack of alternatives. Few women are in decision-making positions in the polity or the economy, making women dependent on men's decisions. A woman cannot afford to demand her rights or to walk off the job if she is treated like an inferior. She will be treated like an inferior everywhere else, and like an unemployed inferior to boot.

Thus the limitations on women's opportunities everywhere else make it possible for the health service industry to offer low wages for high skills and to keep women down. The outside limitations lead women to accept subordination within health service. Health service, at least, is an area in which they can get skills, get jobs, and have the self-respect of making an important contribution to society.

MAINTAINING THE SYSTEM

Health service, then, has a sex hierarchy as well as an occupational hierarchy. The decision makers are almost entirely males and the workers are largely female. It is generally assumed that women as workers are satisfied with their positions in both hierarchies within the industry, that women workers will not fight for their economic welfare as men would, and that as women they accept the leadership of the male sex. The assumption is false.

The labor force pattern of women is now changing. More women are able to continue working despite childbearing, or to drop out for shorter periods of time. More women have a long career ahead of them, and they are increasingly in a position to demand the opening of high-level positions to them (5). Women now fight for position when they can. The modern health service industry has been permeated with internal economic conflict since it began, and the conflicts have grown as the industry has expanded.

To understand the peculiar nature of some of the conflicts in health service, we should examine the way the system is maintained. Health service is somewhat like the construction industry in having separate specialized crafts, with work performed on a custom basis in a large number of small work units (15, 16). Each health occupation above the unskilled level has a separate training program and special entry procedures, often culminating in registration or licensing procedures. Each occupation has a national professional society which tries to function like a craft union.

Unlike the construction industry, however, many highly skilled health occupations are relatively low paying and dead-end. In addition, the "crafts" are not independent of each other; they are hierarchically organized with rigid barriers between levels. The top male occupation—physician—controls the female occupations, not only on the job but in the educational programs. The American Medical Association and its affiliate medical societies have the right to set the curriculum, direct the training programs, control professional certification, and sit on the state licensing boards of (at last count) 16 other occupations. Through the Joint Commission for Accreditation of Hospitals, the American Association of Medical Colleges, the American Hospital Association, American Medical Association (AMA), and the Commission on Medical Education, for example, physicians can decide to create new occupations and control the division of labor. In the dental area the American Dental Association controls dental hygienists, assistants, and technicians. Bullough (17) has shown that historically the development of medicine as an elite profession depended on the patronage of socially powerful institutions external to health service, such as universities. This continues to be true. State legislatures, federal funders, government regulators, college and university administrators, and others support the power of physicians to control other occupations through, for example, hospital staffing regulations, Medicare funding regulations, rights of accreditation, and licensing laws (18).

The nursing profession has escaped total medical control only by its self-conscious determination to be an independent profession, yet organized nursing has far less power in the health service industry than one would expect of an occupation of so many workers and so key to the industry. The American Nursing Association (ANA) and the National League for Nursing (NLN) are generally ignored by the health service industry elite and its outside supporters on questions of public policy with respect to health care. The ANA and the NLN have no voice on the Joint Commission for Accreditation of Hospitals in regulating occupations and hospitals. On the job, nurses are very much subordinate to doctors. Although some of the middle-ranking occupations assert some controls over lower-ranking occupations following the physicians' model, they cannot assert power because they have little or none to assert (see below).

The formal controls on occupations are reinforced by the personal relations between employers and employees, superiors and subordinates at the work site. Who is allowed to work and who is allowed to make decisions are controlled by the same interlocking mechanisms explained above.

Both the ranking system and the ranks of each individual are as obvious in hospitals as in the armed forces. The individual's position is identified by distinctive uniforms and name tags which list occupation and department. As in the armed forces, a superior rank carries weight across departments—a physician on one medical service can often endanger the job of a technician or assistant on another service. Since jobs are insecure, everyone knows not to cross a superior, even though many acts of arrogance or unfairness in superiors can be traced to sexism or racism rather than to mere bureaucratic superiority. Those who complain fear being charged with insubordination, bad work attitudes, or disrespect to the superior.

In case individuals might begin with bad attitudes, training programs for the subordinate occupations include "professional ethics," in which they are taught primarily how to respect the physician and be loyal members of "the team." One chief radiologic technologist at a training hospital complained to this author that the radiologic technologists allow themselves to be pushed around by the doctors, but then he said ruefully, "But I suppose it is our own fault—that's what we teach them to do in the ethics courses."

To a certain extent teaching such "ethics" is unnecessary. Individual placements in the occupational hierarchy reflect the placements in the social hierarchy—men over women, whites over non-whites—and each has spent a lifetime learning how to act toward the other. When an intern is coached on how to handle nurses to get what he wants (19) he is simply relearning at a higher level his teenage lessons on how to handle girls.

The overlap between occupational and sexual status is so great it is sometimes hard to tell which is which. If a male physiologist ignores a female physical therapist's suggestion, is this because the physical therapist knows less, or because women don't know anything worth listening to? When she does not make the suggestion in the first place, has she learned her ethics as a physical therapist or has she learned her place as a woman? When a black nurses' aide talks back to a white nurse, is she being an uppity nurses' aide or is she being an uppity black?

Lest we think that the bureaucratic hierarchy is the primary reason for the superior-subordinate interaction, let us consider what happens when the two hierarchies do not overlap.

Nurses know how to respond to doctors because women know how to respond to men. But what if the doctor is a woman or the nurse a man? Suppose in our previous example the physiologist were a woman and the physical therapist a man? Suddenly the standardized behaviors that were presumed to flow from occupational hierarchies are thrown into turmoil. Much of the "natural" behaviors between occupations turn out to be based on the sex of the incumbent rather than the status of the occupation. Male doctors do not treat male subordinates the same way they treat female subordinates (20). Studies of female doctors show that they often try to identify with their occupational superiority and are perceived as "arrogant" in trying to get the same assistance from nurses and other women subordinates that the men get automatically (21, 22). Similar problems arise when a women chief technician runs a partly male department, or a black therapist supervises white therapy aides. Male orderlies often resent orders given by female nurses. The behavior patterns seen in hospitals between women and men of different occupations are very much sex-status patterns, just as the interpersonal relations between blacks and whites of different occupations are racial relations.

CONFLICTS

While it would appear that male physicians and hospital administrators have the upper hand through their ability to control other occupations, their ability to go outside the system for support, and the deference imposed on subordinates, the apparently iron-clad control system does not necessarily work. Women do fight for opportunities, and have most commonly followed the physicians' model of a professional society fighting for the status of its members.

Because occupational and sexual segregation overlap, conflict often revolves around the shape and structure of the occupations and can best be characterized as maneuvering for "turf"—for control of occupational territory.

Historically, physicians fought hard to suppress midwifery, and by World War Two finally won for physicians the right to deliver babies (23). Now general practitioners are being prevented from assisting at hospital deliveries by obstetricians. Both general practitioners and obstetricians have fought against public health nurses and nurse-midwives giving service in rural areas and urban slums, but this fight presents a dilemma for physicians. Maternity, like most medical specialties, is on a fee-for-service basis. Obstetricians may want to assure that they alone have the right to the fee for this service, but few want the reciprocal obligation of giving the service where there is no fee to be gained. As a result, there is an appallingly high maternal death rate from lack of medical care. Nurse-midwives, after years of struggle, have gained "permission," we might say, to become the inexpensive substitute for the expensive private practitioners, but only in the rural and urban areas that obstetricians do not want (24). Organized medicine keeps a careful watch to see that nurse-midwifery does not expand into serving the more affluent population. Nurse-midwifery services are as yet a controlled threat to a lucrative medical specialty (25). Similarly, nurse-anesthetists are a real threat to anesthesiologists, who have attempted without success to abolish the occupation (26).

The nursing profession has developed other clinical specialists whose skills and training with that specialty are greater than the average physician's, and who can undercut the physician-specialists' high wage rates. Physicians on their part attempt to undercut the threat of nurse specialists by creating lower-skilled substitutes such as obstetrical technicians and operating room assistants who are under AMA control and physicians' authority.

The occupation of licensed practical nurse (LPN) or licensed vocational nurse was consciously created over the objections of the nursing profession by physicians in medical schools and university-affiliated hospitals, who sought a less-trained, lower-paid, and more controllable alternative to the registered nurse, and the LPN was quickly accepted by hospitals and state licensing boards for the same reasons (3). The nursing profession was not able to prevent the development of the LPN, but was able to incorporate LPNs into the National League for Nursing structure and to obtain some control over licensing. Simultaneously with the LPN movement the three-year registered nurse programs were terminated in hospitals and two-year community college programs were created, although the nursing profession favored and has developed four-year B.S. training for nurses (27, 28).

With the shortage of physicians and the high cost of care by physicians, nurses began to develop nurse-practitioners, thus moving into the physicians' territory of diagnosing and curing. Physicians countered with the physician assistant, an occupation completely controlled by physicians, as nurses are not. The occupation was first advertised as a means by which physicians in private practice could increase their patient load and boost their incomes by letting someone else do the work. In this it was similar to the development by dentists of the dental assistant and dental hygienist occupations. The physician assistants were intended to be on a higher level than mere nurses—better paid and possessing medical skills and some decision-making power, but functioning only under the control and direction of physicians (29). They were also intended to be men, especially Vietnam-veteran medics. However, men are expensive and not automatically respectful of the physician's male status, and men can get better-paying, more responsible jobs elsewhere. The physician assistant programs are now primarily training women, taking the same amount of time as nurses' training, and currently at issue is whether physician assistants, standing *in loco medicus,* can give orders to nurses or whether nurses, as independent professionals, can give orders to physician assistants (30).

The sex identification of the occupations is an important component in many of the struggles. Physicians attempt to stamp out lower-level male professions such as podiatrist and optometrist, and attempt to develop women's occupations that can be controlled. Since women have little social power, men are assured of their own primacy. In any other industry a professional society or union which represents half the workers would not be as blithely ignored as is the ANA. Governments and educators simply do not pay attention to mere women. Although 40 per cent of medical technologists are men, the American Society of Medical Technologists (ASMT) is collectively referred to by the clinical pathologist leadership as "the girls." The organization is treated as men treat women—as not very serious and not needing to be taken into account when decisions are made that affect them. When the ASMT elected its first male president, one prominent woman technologist wondered if the ASMT would now be called "the girls and boys."

The pathologists' belief in women's collective subordination has backfired, as did belief in the collective subordination of nurses. The men might not wish to take the women seriously, but the women find their situation to be no laughing matter. Conflict in laboratory technology is rampant (31).

Although medical technologists, with college graduation and a year of clinical training behind them, are the official subordinate profession in pathology laboratories, pathologists have hired lower-paid technicians, usually with a year or two of college and no formal training. To protect themselves, the medical technologists attempted to create an occupation subordinate to themselves in the laboratory assistant, a high school graduate with one year of training who was intended to squeeze out technicians. The pathologists, however, refused to sponsor that level. Desiring a less troublesome but still skilled assistant occupation, the pathologists began to develop an official technician program, requiring two years of college and one year of training, which the technologists refused to sponsor. Pathologists subsequently sought tighter control over technologists' schools and registration. Technologists then sued the pathologists as a combination in restraint of trade. The best efforts of the AMA and out-of-court mediators have not brought a satisfactory solution. The ASMT has begun developing master's degrees in laboratory management, an area the pathologists consider to be their exclusive prerogative, and the American Society of Clinical Pathologists has withdrawn some financial support from ASMT and its related organizations.

INDUSTRIALISM

The change to hospitals and clinics as the first line of medical defense has weakened the independent power of physicians, who no longer control the market. The AMA's lessened influence on national medical policy is indicative of this. Increasing financial involvement of government, insurance companies, and other corporations has inevitably brought increased power to those institutions at the expense of hospital administrators as well as physicians (32). These third parties, as they are known in the trade, are not as interested in supporting the status quo as in providing inexpensive, efficient, and often profitable health service.

This increasing industrialization will clearly restructure the health occupational system, although if it follows current trends the structuring will be downward. Lesser-skilled and lesser-paid subordinates will replace the higher-skilled, higher-paid subordinates, just as the semi-skilled factory workers have replaced craftsmen in other industries. The current rigid occupational structure does enable women to retain some exclusive occupational territory and to attempt to move up by group mobility into the higher slots. However, the rigid segregation produced the high-skilled, low-paid, dead-end nature of health work in the first place. The likelihood of success through this strategy is questionable.

Other changes may be more productive of upward mobility. Clinics, hospitals, and Health Maintenance Organizations are now increasingly replacing the private physician even in formerly lucrative areas, and physicians more and more are adopting the role of backup personnel and paid staff rather than that of controllers of medical care. The administrative side of medicine then becomes more important, and produces a different potential for the lower occupations.

For one thing, the physician loses the personal incentive to keep down the training and wages of subordinates as he had in private practice. Since the wages are being paid by hospitals rather than by the physician, the physician wants the best assistants money can buy. Hospital-based physicians sometimes side with the upwardly mobile women's occupations against the hospital administrators and private practitioners (33).

In addition, most physicians have not perceived administration as a career ladder to success or as a major means to industrial power.[1] Members of subordinate occupations are developing hierarchies within their occupations and are moving upward there and in the administrative hierarchy. This permits them a certain amount of occupational self-control and even some bureaucratic control over the practice of physicians. The subordinate occupations are taking steps to enhance mobility by writing administrative positions into their own staffing guides, adding management courses to their training programs, and adding articles about administration to their professional society journals.

However, these new bureaucratic opportunities tend to benefit the men and the whites within the lower occupations more than they benefit the women and blacks.

---

[1] A past governor of the American College of Surgeons perceives the development as follows: "Nurses originated as helpers for doctors but over the years they have assumed more and more administrative functions until they occupy a position midway between administrative and professional staff. Many doctors regret this development but it has come about because of the laissez-faire attitude of doctors so that they have no real basis for complaint. As long as nurses realize and remember their primary mission of assisting the doctor in the care of his patients, no real harm results" (34).

Lower-level administrators are appointed from above and the top tends to choose its own kind. For example, chief radiologic technologists, who are promoted by administration, are twice as likely to be men as are radiologic technologists as a whole. The form of the stratification may change, but the membership composition by race and sex at each level may remain the same. As long as control flows from the top down, and the top is a small minority of white males in a system that fosters racism and sexism, the relative positions of white men, non-white men, white women, and non-white women will (or may) remain the same.

UNIONISM

As the private office and small hospital are replaced by the large hospital and clinic, there is not only an increasing number of occupations, but also an increased number of workers within each occupation, in national communication with each other. Health service has become a major form of employment. These are the ideal conditions for unionization. Both craft unionism, in which workers are organized by occupation, and industrial unionism, where workers are organized by employing unit, have increased (35).

Nurses' strikes are an example of what craft unionism can accomplish (36, 37). This kind of militance is only possible when there are enough members of an occupation in positions that can bring the hospitals to a halt. Hospital technicians on both the east and west coasts, mostly male, have attempted similar unionism and have largely failed, because their numbers are too small and the skills can be bought elsewhere. Nurses' strikes are aided not only by sufficient strength and number but also by the militance that the subordinate position of women can create. Having no future to lose, they can risk a strike, and they are brought together by their mutual identity as women as well as nurses. In addition, nurses who have carefully developed the identity of nursing as a profession giving service to patients are outraged by their treatment as assembly-line workers giving skilled labor to employers.

Industrial unionism is typified by hospital strikes, in which all the employees of one hospital or one city's hospitals are organized as a unit. Such organizing is aided by the development of large medical centers employing hundreds and even thousands of low-paid workers (38).

There is tremendous hostility to strikes in the health sector, in part because strikes interfere with treatment but in part because of the sex and often race of the striking workers. The enormous hostility to the hospital workers' strike in New York City in the early 1960s resulted in large part from the fact that the strikers were mostly non-whites and women and identified themselves with the civil rights struggle. "How dare they?" would best characterize the response of hospital administrators and the informed public. Similar upper-level sentiment against the San Francisco nurses' strikes was outrage that women would do such things. The California Nurses Association sees its struggle as a woman's struggle. In many cases, hospital strikers realize that their problems within the work setting are based partly on their sex and race status in the community (39).

Although people can unite around their sexual and racial oppression, these factors can also hold back organization, as can the segregation of occupations (40). Workers often feel more solidarity with their occupational colleagues in other hospitals than they do with their fellow workers in their own hospital, some of whom are in competing occupations and some of whom are of occupations, races, or sex perceived as inferior.

Strikes have failed because white strikers ignored black workers and black strikers ignored white workers, or because of male-female hostility. All these differences are exploited by the upper level. One major hospital union was not able to organize the nurses, technicians, and therapists into an industrial union until they developed a separate professional guild for these higher-level workers. In one hospital I studied which was undergoing a unionism drive, a technician explained her opposition to the union with, "Why should I have to go on strike because a porter throws a broom against a wall?" This same argument was given me by the laboratory administrator as a reason "his girls" should not join the union, leaving me with a strong impression about where the argument originated. The objection to the porter was not merely occupational. All of the porters who might have thrown their brooms against the wall were black men; all the technicians were white women. Thus race, sex, and professionalism combined against the union.

Professionalism is often seen as the antithesis of unionism and is used in this way. Said the chairman of the radiologists' Committee on Technician Affairs (41):

> Better trained and better paid technologists have a more professional attitude and are less likely to seek unionization and licensing as solutions for their problems. They also more properly appreciate their role in medicine and their relationship to their radiologists.

Nevertheless, in the attempt to push away unions, the professional societies are themselves having to respond to the rising demands of their members, and have taken actions resembling those of unions, partially in fear that their members will desert them in favor of unions. The radiologic technologists instituted a salary study "to meet head-on the encroachment of unionization. . . ."(42). The resulting salary proposals were so far above prevailing wage rates as to resemble nothing so much as the bargaining demands of a union.

Unionism seems promising, and hospital unions have been successful in raising the wages and bargaining position of hospital workers across occupational, race, and sex lines, and many have been making efforts to open mobility channels for low-level workers. However, unionism as a whole in this country has been both racist and sexist and has tended to become subordinate to management. If unions are to solve the problems, women must have power within them (43). The unions must remain aware of the need for equality for women and non-whites, and aware of the need to challenge management's right to rule.

CONCLUSION

A successful struggle against sexism in health service, as against racism, requires the unification of women and non-whites at all occupational levels in a common struggle not only against particular hospitals or occupations but against the entire structure of the health service industry that sustains low wages for the majority of workers and poor quality of care for the general population.

REFERENCES

1. Weiss, J. The Changing Job Structure of Health Manpower. Unpublished dissertation, Harvard University, Cambridge, 1966.
2. National Center for Health Statistics. *Health Resources Statistics: Health Manpower and Health Facilities 1971.* U.S. Department of Health, Education, and Welfare, 1972.
3. Reverby, S. Health: Women's work. *Health-PAC Bulletin* 40: 1-3, April 1972.
4. Rosenberg, M. *Occupations and Values.* Free Press, Glencoe, Ill., 1957.
5. Kreps, J. *Sex in the Marketplace.* Johns Hopkins Press, Baltimore, 1971.
6. Oppenheimer, V. K. *The Female Labor Force in the United States.* Population Monograph Series No. 5, University of California, Berkeley, 1970.
7. Greenfield, H. I., with Brown, C. A. *Allied Health Manpower: Trends and Prospects.* Columbia University Press, New York, 1969.
8. Women's Bureau. *Handbook on Women Workers.* U.S. Department of Labor, 1969.
9. Women's Bureau. *Facts about Women Workers.* U.S. Department of Labor, 1974.
10. Flaim, P. O., and Peters, N. I. Usual weekly earnings of American workers. *Monthly Labor Review* 95(3): 28-38, 1972.
11. Bureau of the Census. *General Social and Economic Characteristics, United States Summary, 1970.* U.S. Department of Commerce, 1972.
12. Mitchell, J. *Woman's Estate.* Pantheon, New York, 1972.
13. Ladinsky, J. Occupational determinants of geographic mobility among professional workers. *Amer. Sociol. Rev.* 32: 253-264, April 1967.
14. Smith, P. D. *Influence of Wage Rates on Nurse Mobility.* Graduate Program in Hospital Administration, University of Chicago, Chicago, 1962.
15. Kissick, W. *Health Manpower in Transition.* U.S. Public Health Service, 1966.
16. Coggeshall, L. T. *Planning for Medical Progress through Education.* Association of American Medical Colleges, Evanston, Ill., April 1965.
17. Bullough, V. L. *The Development of Medicine as a Profession.* S. Karger, Basel and New York, 1966.
18. Spieler, E. Division of laborers. *Health-PAC Bulletin* 46: 1-2, 4, November 1972.
19. Nolen, W. A. *The Making of a Surgeon.* Simon and Schuster, New York, 1972.
20. Cooper, V. The lady's not for burning. *Health-PAC Bulletin* pp. 2-3. March 1970.
21. Lopate, C. *Women in Medicine.* Johns Hopkins Press, Baltimore, 1968.
22. Kosa, J., and Cocker, R. E., Jr. The female physician in public health: Conflict and reconciliation of the sex and professional roles. *Sociology and Social Research* 49(3): 294-305, 1965.
23. Ehrenreich, B., and English, D., editors. *Witches, Midwives, and Nurses: A History of Women Healers.* Feminist Press, Old Westbury, New York, 1973.
24. *The Training and Responsibilities of the Midwife.* The Josiah Macy Jr. Foundation, New York, 1967.
25. *The Midwife in the United States,* Josiah Macy Jr. Foundation, New York, 1968.
26. Stevens, R. *American Medicine and the Public Interest.* Yale University Press, New Haven, 1971.
27. Levine, E. Some answers to the nurse shortage. *Nursing Outlook* 12(3): 30-34, 1964.
28. Levine, E., Siegel, S., and De La Prente, J. Diversity of nurse staffing among general hospitals. *Hospitals* 35(9): 42-48, 1961.
29. Lippard, V., and Purcell, E., editors. *Intermediate-Level Health Practitioners.* Josiah Macy Jr. Foundation, New York, 1973.
30. Reverby, S. Sorcerer's apprentice. *Health-PAC Bulletin* 46: 1-2, November 1972.
31. Brown, C. A. The division of laborers: Allied health professions. *Int. J. Health Serv.* 3(3): 435-444, 1973.
32. Ehrenreich, B., and Ehrenreich, J. *The American Health Empire: Power, Profits and Politics.* Random House, New York, 1970.
33. Brown, C. A. The Development of Occupations in Health Technology. Unpublished dissertation, Columbia University, New York, 1971.
34. Bowers, W. F. *Interpersonal Relationships in the Hospital.* Charles C Thomas, Springfield, Ill., 1960.
35. Gershenfeld, W. J. Labor Relations in Hospitals. Paper presented at Emerging Sectors of Collective Bargaining Seminar No. 4, Temple University, Philadelphia, March 28, 1968.
36. The male-feasance of health. *Health-PAC Bulletin,* March 1970.

37. Gaynor, D., Blake, E., Bodenheimer, T., and Mermey, C. RN strike: Between the lines. *Health-PAC Bulletin* 60: 1-2, 5, September-October 1974.
38. Davis, L. State of the Union. *1199 Drug and Hospital News,* pp. 20-23, March 1969.
39. Institutional organizing. *Health-PAC Bulletin* No. 37, January 1972.
40. Fragmentation of workers: An anti-personnel weapon. *Health-PAC Bulletin* No. 46, November 1972.
41. Soule, A. B. Trends in training programs in radiologic techology. *Radiol. Technol.* 38: 70-73, 1966.
42. Proceedings of the thirty-ninth annual convention. *Radiol. Technol.* 39: 98, September 1967.
43. Bergquist, V. A. Women's participation in labor unions. *Monthly Labor Review* 97(10): 3-9, 1974.

CHAPTER 12

Barriers To The Nurse Practitioner Movement: Problems Of Women In A Woman's Field

Bonnie Bullough

While it is obvious that women who break the sex barrier to enter fields previously dominated by men have problems related to their sex, the problems of a woman in a woman's field are less apparent. It is, however, still possible to suffer from sex discrimination in an occupation like nursing which is more than 98 per cent female. Nursing, in fact, is a good example of a profession which has lived with sex barriers, learned to cope with them, and now finds that those very coping mechanisms are blocking progress. This can be seen most clearly when the barriers to the nurse practitioner movement are examined. Nurses now are expanding their scope of practice to take on new responsibilities, but for a time it looked as if this would not be possible because of psychological and legal barriers created by past subordination and by the nurses' own response to that subordination. In fact, the impetus for the expanding role is largely due to forces outside nursing.

One of the major factors causing expansion was the shortage of primary care physicians. Originally this shortage resulted from an increased demand for health care even though the number of medical school graduates each year had remained virtually constant for more than 50 years (1). Although the number of physicians is now increasing slightly, the increase has been more than offset by the trend toward specialization; specialists now outnumber general practitioners by more than three to one (2). The result has been to create a gap in the health care delivery system which must be filled by other workers.

NURSE PRACTITIONERS VERSUS PHYSICIAN ASSISTANTS

Until recently it seemed that the most likely candidates for filling this need would be the physician assistants rather than nurse practitioners. These young men are chosen from the ranks of independent duty corpsmen who have been discharged from the armed services and who are given up to two years of additional training before being

127

sent out as assistants to busy physicians (3, 4). They have received much favorable coverage in the public as well as the medical press.

There are, however, some disadvantages to the physician assistant approach. The supply of discharged independent duty corpsmen is limited, particularly now that the nation is changing over to a peacetime army, and some of the training programs have been forced to consider other candidates. In contrast, there are approximately 800,000 employed registered nurses in the country (5), all of whom have at least a high school diploma and most of whom have considerable additional academic preparation. The basic training for corpsmen varies from one branch of the service to another but is usually about ten weeks. The independent duty corpsman augments this training with a correspondence course or occasionally by formal classroom work, but the extra training seldom lasts more than one year. The minimum training for a registered nurse is two years, with many of the nurse practitioner programs requiring that their candidates also hold baccalaureate degrees. Thus the nurses have better backgrounds than the corpsmen in the physical, biological, and social sciences as well as the actual techniques of health care before they enter the special nurse practitioner courses which last from 4 to 18 months.

Because of these factors the nurse practitioner movement is at last gaining momentum. Since 1971, 21 states have revised their nurse practice acts to facilitate role expansion for nurses into the area of diagnosis and treatment and other states are expected to join this movement (6). The estimated 10,000 nurse practitioners presently in the field include pediatric, geriatric, adult, maternity, and family nurse practitioners (7). In addition, 1,500 nurse-midwives have been certified by the American College of Nurse-Midwifery (8), bringing the number of practitioners to a significantly greater total than the total of 900 physician assistants as estimated in 1973 (9).

With all of these advantages it is reasonable to ask why the nurses did not preempt the field from the beginning. Why did they stand by and allow a new occupation to develop to fill a need which nurses, with only a minimum amount of additional training, could easily fill? The answers to these questions are somewhat complex and are grounded in the fact that most registered nurses are women, whereas the corpsmen are men.

Nursing, probably more than any occupation except housewifery and prostitution, reflects the stereotyped role of women. The norms and values of nursing are feminine and the relationships between nurses and physicians reflect the extreme subordination of women with all of the male-female games which tend to go along with that subordination. Moreover, the educational system has, at least in the past, tended to reinforce this feminine and subordinate role of the nurse and new generations of students have been taught to be "ladylike," subservient, and manipulative.

HISTORICAL REASONS FOR THE SUBORDINATION OF NURSES

There are some historical reasons for this feminine image of nursing and the subordination to the physician, but the historical precedents are not as ancient as many people believe. While it is true that throughout our history most sick people were cared for in their homes by unpaid relatives and that usually these home nurses were women, many of the professional nurses in the past were men. The priests in the Greek Temples of Aesculapius who gave nursing care were men. Most of the battlefield nursing was done by men. One of the reasons the Romans were able to extend their conquests so far was the fact that they were able to minimize losses on the battlefield by setting up first aid procedures and caring for their wounded in movable tent hospitals rather than leaving them to die as many other ancient armies did. The nurse (or tent companion, as he was called) became a specialist in the Roman legions (10).

During the medieval period there were several all-male monastic nursing orders, such as the Knights Templars and the Lazarists, although in the later middle ages female orders became much more numerous and the occupation of nursing, as differentiated from home nursing, became more female-oriented. Increasingly, as women moved into the field the status of the occupation fell, and two types of nurses developed: religious sisters who were respected for their vows of poverty, chastity, and obedience, and secular nurses who were classed with the lowest level of servants (10, pp. 30-36). These two divisions were successfully merged in the middle of the 19th century by Florence Nightingale, who helped to bring the aura of the religious order to secular nursing, but in the process the sex segregation of the occupation grew more pronounced.

The Role of Florence Nightingale

Nightingale was a brilliant woman whose achievements in establishing nursing schools, in research, and in reforming the British army were monumental. However, her major achievement was probably that of an image-maker who established secular nursing as a respectable occupation for women. Her work as a nurse at Scutari during the Crimean War was reported in great detail by the British press and it made her a heroine to the mass of people. Unfortunately for today's nurses, however, Florence Nightingale never worked directly. She was a master manipulator who was able to get other people, usually men, to speak for her while she pretended helplessness. In Scutari, although she came with significant power delegated to her by the Secretary of War, she refused to allow the nurses under her command to give any care to the suffering men until the surgeons "ordered" them to do so. This mechanism gained her the support of the army doctors, who were very suspicious of her as well as the 38 nurses who came with her, but it also helped establish the surgeon as superior to the nurse (11).

After the war Florence Nightingale started her monumental work of reforming the army to secure better pay and more humane treatment for the common soldier. She accomplished this reform in a ladylike, although unique, fashion. She retired from public view and withdrew gradually into seclusion until she finally simply took to her bed, where she stayed for the last 50 years of her life. Sitting in her bed she wrote letters, collected data, and drafted lengthy, well documented position papers, but she never appeared in public to defend these positions. Instead, she convinced her various male friends and admirers (including Sidney Herbert, a former Secretary of War), that they should present her arguments to Parliament and wage the public fight for reform. She claimed that she was a weak, feeble woman, and the work of public struggles should be handled by great strong men (11, pp. 162-366). While this method was probably the key to her effectiveness, the precedent which she set for women and nurses has not been without negative consequences.

In 1860, Nightingale used funds which had been raised to honor her to set up the famous nursing school at St. Thomas' Hospital. As the news of the school spread, people from around the world traveled to her bedside to seek advice on how to set up similar "Nightingale" schools in their hospitals, as well as to get hints on how to better run their hospitals or district nursing services. Her mark on nursing was indelible. She insisted that nurses should be clean, chaste, quiet, and religious. She agreed with hospital authorities that nurses should work long hours, never complain, and be obedient to their superiors and physicains. She was against any self-determination on the part of nurses and fought against the organization of the British Nurses Association. She argued that good character was more important than knowledge in producing a good nurse, so the Nightingale model in nursing education stressed apprenticeship training in the simple procedures, with long hours and stringent rules to help the students avoid temptation (10, pp. 107-113).

It is of course an oversimplification to lay all of the blame for the subordination of nurses on Florence Nightingale, just as it is an oversimplification to accuse Sigmund Freud of subordinating 20th-century housewives. Both of these people were 19th-century figures who were great innovators in their own specialty, but they adhered to traditional Victorian beliefs about the proper role and status of women. This is true of Florence Nightingale even though she helped create a work role for women which took them outside of the home; the nursing role was shaped in a completely traditional manner and the accepted interaction patterns of the sexes were not disturbed. Since Nightingale and Freud were innovators only within the context of their times, it would be unfair to complain about the blind spots exhibited by these 19th-century figures. The real culprits are their 20th-century followers, who have uncritically accepted the more repressive assumptions along with the positive contributions.

HOSPITAL TRAINING SCHOOLS

The major social structure which institutionalized and perpetuated the 19th century subordination of nurses was the hospital training school. The two primary functions of the modern hospital are to assist physicians in their practice of medicine and to serve patients who are ill (12). Thus when American hospital nursing schools were established their goal was clearly one of service rather than one of education, in contrast to a college or university. Nurse training schools were opened to improve patient care and to save money; educating students was seen as a method for achieving these objectives but certainly not as a goal in and of itself. Student nurses in this period were expected to work long hours and were allowed to hear lectures only when it would not interfere with their ward duties (10, pp. 148-180; 13).

Because the educational process was primarily by apprenticeship, nurses learned by doing, although eventually more class work was added to the curriculum as graduate nurses pressed for reform. The student was considered the lowest person in the status hierarchy and was responsible for much of the work now done by aides and janitors, as well as for patient care. Students were answerable to members of the hospital administrative hierarchy, physicians, and teachers (if separate teachers were hired). The physician was considered the most significant of these three and was such an awesome authority figure that, until about 20 years ago, student nurses were taught to stand up when a doctor entered the room and to open the door for all men because most men in the hospital environment at that time were physicians. Although these might be considered harmless symbols of subordination (unless the nurse accidently tripped over a man who was attending to the norms of the broader society and opening the door for a woman), a distinctly harmful aspect of the extreme subordination which students were taught was the intellectual subordination. A cornerstone of the hospital nursing school education was a belief that the physician was always right, and even when he was wrong he must be made to appear right.

This system tended to exclude the rebels and the serious scholars who had other alternatives for an education, including most of the men. According to census figures, 7 per cent of the working nurses in 1910 were men, and that figure probably represents a decline from earlier decades (10, p. 205); only 1.4 per cent of the registered nurses are now men (5, p. 7). The men who did not exclude themselves were often excluded by the hospital schools on the grounds of a housing problem. In the tradition of live-in servants as well as to protect their morals, student nurses were required to live in a dormitory called a nurses' home. The norms of the day and the high moral stance of the schools precluded men from living in the nurses' home, and the lower status of student nurses precluded their being housed in the interns' quarters. Thus, to avoid the problem, men were often simply not admitted to the schools. The few men who did graduate in the first half of the 20th century came primarily from a few all-male nursing schools (10, p. 205).

EDUCATIONAL REFORM

Eventually educational reform did come to nursing, but only after a long and painful struggle. Although the first collegiate school was opened at the University of Minnesota in 1909 (14), the hospitals were reluctant to give up the valuable free help they received from the student nurses and the university intellectual communities questioned admitting nurses. A whole series of national reports were issued recommending that, for the good of the nation as well as the profession, nursing education should be transferred from the hospitals to educational institutions (13, 15-17), but change came so slowly that a half-century after the foundation of the Minnesota program only 16 per cent of the new nurses were graduated from a basic program which was operated by an educational institution (18).

Probably the most significant development promoting change has been the recent growth of the community college movement. Since these community or junior colleges are vocationally oriented they are less reluctant to accept nurses and are rapidly becoming the major source of basic nursing education. In 1972, for the first time in the history of American nursing education, there were more nurses graduated from collegiate than diploma programs, with 37 per cent of the new graduates finishing associate of arts programs, 21 per cent receiving baccalaureate degrees, and 42 per cent graduating from hospital diploma schools (5, pp. 70-71). Moreover, the competition has forced the hospital diploma programs to hire adequate teaching staffs and cut hours worked by students to only those needed for clinical learning, so it is now expensive rather than profitable to run a nursing school and most of the diploma programs have seriously considered the possibility of terminating. Nursing education is finally moving into the mainstream of American higher education.

CURRENT ATTITUDES AS BARRIERS TO ROLE EXPANSION

However, the weight of past tradition, the subordination of nurses, the sex segregation, and the apprenticeship model in nursing education have left a mark on the attitudes of present day nurses. As the programs moved into the colleges and universities the curriculums were strengthened, but for a time the emphasis, particularly in the bachelor's degree programs, was placed on giving emotional support to the ill patient rather than on diagnosing or treating his presenting complaint. The supporters of this approach felt that the patient care role should be divided into "care" and "cure" components, with nurses giving psychosocial support and physicians carrying full responsibility for the diagnosis and treatment of the patient. This division was defended partly in an effort to find an independent niche for nurses but also because nurses were felt to be more naturally maternal and expressive than physicians. This philosophy has acted as a major deterrent to the development of the nurse practitioner role, which contains both care and cure components, and it remains the focus of disagreement among the ranks of nursing educators (19).

There are other nurses who still believe that they cannot and should not take any independent responsibility, or more accurately that they should not be held accountable for their own decisions. They are able to believe this in spite of the fact that much of the time the patient's life depends on the nurse's ability to assess his condition and act intelligently on that assessment. Of course, nurses do not actually avoid all decision making. They merely pretend to avoid it. The shortage of men in the profession and the quota system in medicine which operated for many years to limit the number of women admitted to medical schools made the sex segregation between medicine and nursing an extreme one, and stylized communication patterns have grown up between the two professions. These communication patterns are further distorted by the fact that nurses in hospitals and other institutional settings are also under the control of the administrative hierarchy. Since they must answer to two seemingly absolute and often opposite lines of authority, the administrative and the medical, nurses have been forced to learn to negotiate, and gamesmanship has become a part of their lives (20, 21).

GAMES NURSES PLAY

Most of the games nurses play with physicians are built upon the pretense that all decisions about patient care are made by physicians, which is of course not true if only because the physicians are not present when most care is given. When nurses make major decisions they handle the situation by invoking the name of the doctor to the patient and pretending to the doctor that their idea was his idea. They do this by means of hints, flattery, and feminine wiles rather than by making open statements. Such an approach is not unusual among groups of people who have little formal power; they learn to negotiate power by devious means. For example, oriental wives and grandmothers are renowned for the power they are able to accrue through manipulation. However, the nurse-doctor relationships are remarkable when viewed against the more egalitarian norms of contemporary American society.

One of the best early descriptions of the doctor-nurse game was written by a psychiatrist, Leonard Stein (22). His article was originally prepared for a psychiatric journal but it has been reprinted several times in nursing publications because it points out the games so clearly. Stein was fascinated by the strange way in which nurses make recommendations to physicians and the reciprocal pretense on the part of physicians that nurses never make recommendations; yet, he noted, successful physicians are careful to follow nurses' recommendations. Stein called the pattern a transactional neurosis.

The Doctor-Nurse Game: A Questionnaire

To further investigate these types of games a group of University of California graduate students in the school of nursing studied a sample of 103 hospital nurses and 40 physicians. Using a set of situation questions drawn from the students' own past nursing experiences, they asked the nurses in the sample to choose their most likely response. For example, they were asked the following:

A doctor has written an order which you as a nurse question [as correct]. In the past you have found this M.D. to be very adamant about the appropriateness of his orders and insistent that they be carried out. What would your opening statement be?

_____ (a) Doctor, you have made an error.
_____ (b) Doctor, would you like to check this order?
_____ (c) Doctor, you always write such legible, appropriate orders, but if you have time, I wonder if you would clarify this order?
_____ (d) I'm so dense, I don't understand this order.

None of the sampled nurses selected the first alternative; 56 per cent chose the second, 41 per cent the third, and 3 per cent indicated the last alternative. This same question was reworded for the smaller physician sample. The doctor was asked to assume that he had written an incorrect order and he was to indicate which of the same four approaches he would prefer from the nurse. Eleven per cent chose the first answer, 86 per cent the second, 3 per cent the third, and no one checked the last alternative. When this and the other situation questions were tabulated, it was found that the sample nurses tended to choose indirect responses, which could be thought of as polite but which were also suggestive of a certain amount of feminine gamesmanship. There were no significant differences in the preference of the indirect approach as related to the age of the nurse. On the other hand, more physicians indicated in response to the questionnaire that they would prefer nurses to use direct approaches, and there were significant differences related to age, with older physicians more likely to choose the indirect approaches while the younger ones selected the more direct alternatives (23).

These data reiterate the power of past tradition on present day behavior patterns. The fact that a significant number of younger physicians and some older ones do not want, or at least say they do not want, to be "handled" by nurses in a gamesmanship manner seems to be overlooked by nurses who continue to use indirect methods and games rather than open statements of their opinion about patient care. Of course this type of response is not unknown among other groups. Similar patterns of anticipatory withdrawal are fairly common among minority groups; the ghetto walls are often as well policed from the inside as the outside (24, 25). Feelings of powerlessness and fear of punishment can prevent people from challenging the status quo, and the fact that the fear is based upon former traditions and past punishments rather than present realities is often overlooked.

STATE LAWS AS BARRIERS TO ROLE EXPANSION

A similar type of anticipatory withdrawal occurred at the national level and created a serious barrier to the development of nurse practitioners. Starting in 1938, organized nursing attempted to secure mandatory licensure for nurses in all of the states. These laws specified that only registered and practical nurses would be allowed to give nursing care. A necessary part of such a law is a clear definition of nursing at each of the two levels, and definitions were formulated in this period in several states and enacted into law. Finally in 1955, the American Nurses Association, in an effort to assist nurses in the states, decided to formulate a model nurse practice act. This model was subsequently adopted by 15 states in its exact form and by several others in a modified form (26). The most interesting aspect of this definition, which was clearly written by nurses, is the last line, which states, ". . . The foregoing shall not be deemed to include any acts of diagnosis or prescription of therapeutic or corrective measures" (27).

While this anticipatory withdrawal behavior embodied in the disclaimer certainly avoided any boundary dispute with medicine, it probably was unnecessary. There is no documentary or other evidence that medicine in any way coerced the Association into adding the disclaimer. While nurses in that period did not ordinarily prescribe treatments, they were clearly engaged in diagnostic acts. They observed patients, collected data about their conditions, arrived at decisions, and acted on those decisions to care for their patients. While recent developments in primary and intensive care have greatly expanded the role of nurses in the medical decision-making process, the scope of practice statements enacted in this period at the urging of organized nursing were outdated at the time they were written (28).

A decade later when the nurse practitioner movement appeared, the disclaimers in the state nurse practice acts led many people, including the attorney generals of Arizona (29) and California (30), to conclude that the activities of nurse practitioners were illegal. As a result, revision of the state nurse practice acts is required before the nursing role can be expanded, and while in 21 states these revisions have now been accomplished the task of convincing the legislatures to change the law in 29 more states and four other jurisdictions is not small.

SUMMARY

It has been shown that the doctor-nurse game and the anticipatory withdrawal of nurses at both the microcosmic and macrocosmic levels have created formidable barriers to the nurse practitioner movement. Viewed from the historical and sociological perspectives, the difficulties which nurse practitioners have faced in gaining acceptance are easier to understand. The sex segregation of medicine and nursing and the subordinate role of women in the past helped establish traditions, which when nurtured in the exploitive atmosphere of the hospital training schools created patterns of interaction between nurses and physicians which remain as obstacles to the full use of the talents of both professions.

REFERENCES

1. Fein, R. *The Doctor Shortage: An Economic Analysis.* Brookings Institution, Washington, D.C., 1967.

2. *Health Resources Statistics: Health Manpower and Health Facilities,* p. 183. National Center for Health Statistics, Public Health Services Publication No. 1509, 1972-1973.
3. Stead, E. A. Training and use of paramedical personnel. *New Engl. J. Med.* 277(15): 800-801, 1967.
4. Sadler, A., Sadler, B., and Bliss, A. *The Physician's Assistant: Today and Tomorrow.* Yale University Press, New Haven, 1972.
5. *Facts About Nursing 72-73,* p. 6. American Nurses Association, Kansas City, Missouri, 1974.
6. Bullough, B. The changing state of nurse practice arts, Phase III. In *The Law and the Expanding Nursing Role,* edited by B. Bullough. Appleton-Century-Crofts, New York, in press.
7. Personal communication to National Health Law Program from P. H. Dunkley, Deputy Executive Director, Professional Activities Division, American Nurses Association, August 1974.
8. Olsen, L. The expanded role of the nurse in maternity practice. *Nursing Clinics of North America* 9(3): 459-466, 1974.
9. American Medical Association. *Accredited Educational Programs for the Primary Care Physician,* March 1974.
10. Bullough, V., and Bullough, B. *The Emergence of Modern Nursing,* pp. 21-29. Macmillan Company, London, 1969.
11. Woodham-Smith, C. *Florence Nightingale, 1820-1910,* pp. 98-110. McGraw-Hill Book Company, New York, 1951.
12. Rosen, G. The hospital: Historical sociology of a community institution. In *The Hospital in Modern Society,* edited by E. Freidson, pp. 1-36. Free Press of Glencoe, New York, 1963.
13. Goldmark, J., and the Committee for the Study of Nursing Education. *Nursing and Nursing Education in the United States.* Macmillan Company, New York, 1923.
14. Gray, J. *Education for Nursing: A History of the University of Minnesota School.* University of Minnesota Press, Minneapolis, 1960.
15. *Nursing Schools Today and Tomorrow.* Committee on the Grading of Nursing Schools, New York, 1934.
16. Brown, E. L. *Nursing for the Future.* Russell Sage Foundation, New York, 1948.
17. Lysaught, J. P., and the National Commission for the Study of Nursing and Nursing Education. *An Abstract for Action.* McGraw-Hill Book Company, New York, 1970.
18. *Facts About Nursing: A Statistical Summary, 1970-71,* p. 77. American Nurses Association, New York, 1972.
19. Rogers, M. E. Nursing: To be or not to be? *Nurs. Outlook* 20(1): 42-46, 1972.
20. Strauss, A., Schatzman, L., Ehrlich, D., Bucher, R., and Sabshin, M. The hospital and its negotiated order. In *The Hospital in Modern Society,* edited by E. Freidson, pp. 147-169. Free Press of Glencoe, New York, 1963.
21. Smith, H. L. Two lines of authority: The hospital's dilemma. In *Patients, Physicians and Illness,* edited by E. G. Jaco, pp. 468-469. Free Press, Glencoe, Illinois, 1958.
22. Stein, L. I. The doctor-nurse game. *Arch. Gen. Psychiatry* 16(6): 699-703, 1967.
23. Chaffee, K., Kingstedt, C., Reiss, J., Baron, B., Brady, K., Lee, E., Kyung, H. P., Stuart, I., and Bullough, B. A Study of the Doctor-Nurse Game, unpublished manuscript, 1974.
24. Bullough, B. Alienation in the ghetto. *Am. J. Sociol.* 72(5): 469-478, 1967.
25. Bullough, B. *Social Psychological Barriers to Housing Desegregation.* Special Report No. 2. Housing, Real Estate and Urban Land Studies Program, Los Angeles, 1969.
26. Fogotson, E. H., Roemer, R., Newman, R. W., and Cook, J. L. Licensure of other medical personnel. In *Report of the National Advisory Commission on Health Manpower,* Vol. II, pp. 407-492. U.S. Government Printing Office, Washington, D. C., 1967.
27. A.N.A. board approves a definition of nursing practice. *Am. J. Nurs.* 55(12): 1474, 1955.
28. Bullough, B. The Law and the Expanding Nursing Role. Paper read at the Annual Meeting of the American Public Health Association, New Orleans, 1974.
29. *Arizona Attorney General Opinion No. 71-30,* Aug. 6, 1971.
30. *California Attorney General Opinion No. CV72/187,* Feb. 15, 1973.

CHAPTER 13

Women's Emancipation And Socialism: The Case Of The People's Republic Of Poland

Magdalena Sokolowska

". . . and he said that he would marry no girl who sweated at the workbench like a boy. . . . " (From a letter to the weekly magazine *Przyjaciolka*, 1961)

THE CHOICE OF "MALE" AND "FEMALE" OCCUPATIONS

The division of occupations into those which suit men and those which suit women is not based on any scientific anatomical, physiological, or technological studies. It is public opinion that divides occupations in countries in such a way that sometimes the same job is considered the province of both males and females, depending on the country and the cultural ambience. According to Wrochno (1),

> [In Poland] there is the general conviction that tailoring work, for instance, is a typically female profession. When I was once in Guinea, I visited a clothing factory which produced school smocks for girls. At the sewing machines sat a row of men. When I asked why no women worked there, I was told: "The work is too hard for women." Raising chickens has been the women's domain for hundreds of years in Poland. In Guinea I visited a chicken farm. Not one woman worked there. I asked why. The answer was: "Women are not suited to this work."

When women choose an occupation, the education determined for them by the female image in the general social consciousness plays a decisive role. If women in Poland are more inclined to become nurses than mechanics, it can be attributed to the fact that this attitude has been imprinted on them by the entire process of their personality formation, by their education, and by the influence of their environment. In their parents' houses there is often a male/female division of work, and different requirements are made of daughters than of sons. In the schools as well, young girls often learn in vocational classes something other than what the boys are taught. For a

137

woman to work as a nurse or teacher is perceived as a normal occurrence by young girls. A woman in a technical occupation who works at a hoisting crane is sometimes seen, but that is still a relatively rare and not as yet completely accepted phenomenon.

Today, the profession of physician is considered in Poland as being typically a woman's occupation. Even as long ago as the 1920s and 1930s, almost one-fifth of Polish medical doctors and more than 70 percent of the dentists were women (2). In the first years after World War II, the proportion of women students in medical subjects was at its highest level. In subsequent years the proportions changed, a fact that probably can be attributed to official actions to produce a distribution more evenly balanced by sex in medical studies (Table 1). Nevertheless, in 1968, of those receiving an M.D. degree, 52.4 percent were women and 82.9 percent of those graduating as dentists were women. Today as in the past, women predominate among those entering medical studies. In fact, for the past several years, women have had to obtain higher grades on the admissions test than men because only half the positions are open to them (3).

Table 1 shows that the proportion of women in medicine dropped by half from 1951 to 1967. At the same time, the number of women in technical areas more than doubled. This can be attributed to the previously mentioned actions: restrictions in areas where the number of women was too high, and stimulation in areas where the number was unreasonably low. As a result, the structure of subject areas chosen by women has changed and will probably continue to do so. The spectrum of subjects chosen by women is becoming broader all the time, and, in the process, the subject areas chosen are increasingly at variance with traditional "female" preferences.

Table 1 also shows that the proportion of women has increased in agricultural studies, among others. However, the latest statistics will probably show a drop in this area, as there have been restrictions for several years, just as in medical studies, on the number of women entering agricultural fields at the academic level.

Along with restrictions on accepting women into "feminized" subjects, there has been a disposition to accept a certain percentage into "male" areas. In many subject areas in the secondary schools the number of girls accepted for matriculation was limited several years ago. Systematically, the Ministry of Education, the Education Sections of the People's Councils, unions, and women's organizations have been attempting for several years to change traditional views and to form new ones. The People's Councils support a network of career counseling offices throughout Poland. Special directives obligate school authorities to organize information campaigns and seminars for parents and pupils in their final years of primary school. Trustees of the schools and districts, as well as the labor sections of the People's Councils, ensure that the largest possible number of girls is accepted into schools in the technical subject areas.

If the individual education areas are analyzed, it is shown that there is nothing approaching a uniform distribution of the sexes (4). On the level of the middle vocational school, girls are concentrated primarily in schools and classes that prepare them for service careers (e.g. economics, cooking, merchandising, and health care) or for skilled jobs in the clothing, leather goods, food, and textile industries. A similar feminization can be observed in chemical, fine-mechanical, agricultural, forestry, and

Table 1

Distribution of female students in Polish
higher schools among various subject areas[a]

Subject Area	1950-1951	1966-1967
	%	%
Medicine	30.8	15.1
Technology	6.4	14.8
Agriculture	5.1	8.8
Mathematics and natural sciences	13.9	15.6
Jurisprudence and economics	18.4	20.8
Arts	4.6	2.3
Humanities	20.8	22.6
All students	100.0	100.0

[a]Source, *Women in Poland*, p. xxiii. Central Statistical Office, Warsaw, 1968.

mineralogical fields (over 50 percent girls). A similar process is being carried out in the higher semiprofessional schools called *technika*. Those *technika* which prepare people for service careers as well as for jobs in light industry are almost 100 percent feminized. Also the proportion of girls in fields such as chemistry, geology, transportation, geodesy, and architecture (40-50 percent) is increasing steadily in the *technika*.

Of girls accepted in the *technika* in 1967-1968, 28 percent entered true technical areas and 7 percent agricultural areas. This means that approximately one-third of the young women in Poland today chose "male" occupations. In future years, a further feminization of technical subject areas in schools above the level of the primary school can be expected.

On their own initiative, several branches of industry are carrying out projects expected to encourage young women to learn the appropriate professions. For example, heavy industry began training women several years ago. In 1966 the proportion of female students in middle-level schools of the heavy industry branch was not quite 16 percent, but by 1968, it had risen to 25.8 percent. Most often the women students chose fine-mechanics and the specialty of lathe operator or metal cutting machine operator; they least often chose that of mechanic. In training schools of the machine industry, the specialized area of metal grinder was most attractive to the women students. The electrical professions are completely feminized, especially the production of electric lamps and lighting units, as well as the assembly of semiconductor elements.

In some provinces there are long-range plans for educating young women, for instance, in the province of Katowice. The question of employing women is particularly difficult there because of the predominance of heavy industry. In 1963-1964, about 20 percent of those who graduated from primary school did not continue their education. After the resolution was passed that everyone had to continue his or her education until age 18, this percentage dropped, in 1968-1969, to 2 percent. The province authorities point out that, in order to generalize women's education according to a certain plan as well as to meet the requirement for highly trained groups of workers, binding quotas had to be set up by year for females to be accepted at the "male" schools. That was not popular, either in the factories that require male workers for technical occupations, or among the parents and the young women themselves, who retained prejudices against training in occupations considered manly.

There were also certain difficulties for females in adapting to "male" occupations. A survey carried out in 1968 by the Executive Council of the trade unions at the national level demonstrated the necessity of being more attentive to the young workers in general and to women entering previously "male" occupations in particular. Wherever the women had jobs that corresponded to their qualifications and were given initial help (direction by the foreman, adequate supplies of materials, tools, and technical manuals) and whenever they were rewarded for good work and had a chance for promotion, both sides were satisfied—the factory and the women.

The People's Council of Warsaw has conducted a survey of women who have worked at least one year in "male" professions. The Council wanted to know whether these women believed that women should work in the occupation that they had chosen, whether they felt they were accorded all their rights in the factories as workers, and how other workers rated their work. Those questioned represented different occupational groups such as mechanics, electronics, radio and television, transportation, upholstery, and watchmaking. The results showed that 81 percent of the women had no prejudices against their occupation and believed that women could certainly do that kind of work. Almost half the women described the attitude of their coworkers toward their work as "exactly the same as toward the work of the men"; about 18 percent said they were rated "less critically" than the men. The majority of the women respondents answered affirmatively to the question of whether they were satisfied with their work.

The attempt for years to encourage young women to learn technical jobs has not been without success; these students are becoming increasingly aware that graduates in the traditionally "female" subject areas (such as merchandising and clothing) are having difficulties in finding employment that utilizes those skills. The latest data show that, for example, among the graduates of middle-level professional schools in Warsaw, the percentage of women graduating in the areas of mechanics, electronics, or architecture was three times higher in 1971 than it was three years before. While the electronics schools were overflowing, there were too few graduates of tailoring schools in Warsaw in 1971, and the appropriate factories in the capital had to engage many graduates from other areas to meet their personnel requirements.

According to the Economic Inspector of the Warsaw People's Council, the increase in the number of females learning "male" professions has caused no difficulties. Rather, it was the young women who had graduated in subjects such as chemistry, leather goods, shoemaking, candy making, food, or trade who were causing the problem. Obtaining qualification in many areas of electronics and mechanics and in some areas of construction sometimes affords the chance for speedy employment in a job more closely related to one's qualifications than does training in "stagnant" female areas. The Economic Inspector compiled statistics on the percentage of women with training in a "male" profession who actually entered a job corresponding to the qualifications they had acquired, how many women stayed at these jobs, and how many continued their education in an area other than their original one.

The situation in these subject areas may be compared with that in others. In Warsaw, for example, there is a sharp turn away from the professions of saleswoman and tailor. The exodus from these professions, the tendency to change an educational area that was forced upon them (as is often the case), is perhaps a characteristic occurrence among women who have graduated from middle-level schools, especially in areas where demand on the job market is strong, as this facilitates such a reorientation.

As the number of young women graduating from technical schools increases, so do reports in the press about how these graduates are having difficulty finding jobs. Factories offer only a limited number of positions for women. This cannot be attributed solely to prejudices, but also to the fact that "male" professions in general are better paid than "female" ones, so that there exists a strong competition between men and women in these jobs.

The question of enlarging the proportion of males in the "female" subject areas (e.g. secretarial work, merchandising, cooking, and health care) has been given less attention than the reverse to date. There are, however, signs that indicate that this issue is also being considered in the planning activity by state authorities. In 1971, a 2.5-year school for psychiatric nursing intended primarily for boys was started in Lodz. A press report on this subject reported that there were supposed to be extra points in the entrance examination for being male. The press also wrote in a report entitled "First Signs of a Defeminization of Nursing" that two men also participated in the entrance examination in 1971 for the academic School of Nursing at the newly established Nursing Department of the Medical School in Lublin, the only school of its kind in Central Europe.

THE POSITION OF WOMEN IN THE LABOR FORCE

The postulate of female equality in labor has not yet been realized. Both the disparate rates of pay and the unequal positions of men and women are clear evidence of this.

Disparate Rates of Pay

Although pay rates have risen generally, differences in the pay of men and women have continued as before (5, 6). The average pay of women is more than 30 percent lower than that of men (Table 2).

If it is assumed that the principle of equal pay for equal work in a similar work situation is observed, then the inequality of salary must be attributed to the inequality of work positions. Daily observation, as well as numerous investigations, confirms the interpretation that, in the hierarchy of factories—even in a branch of industry as

Table 2

Monthly pay of male and female white-collar workers
at the level of large firms, in September 1960 and September 1965[a]

Monthly Pay	1960		1965	
in Zlotys	Male	Female	Male	Female
	%	%	%	%
Up to 1000	5.1	17.3	1.5	7.3
1000–1500	20.7	36.6	9.8	25.2
1500–2000	26.6	24.8	19.9	33.1
2000–2500	20.3	7.5	20.6	13.3
Over 2500	27.3	3.8	38.2	10.0

[a]Source, reference 1, p. 121.

completely feminized as the textile industry—men have higher positions of authority than women. In this industry, both in production and in management, there are only a few women in top positions. The differences between the pay of men and women are closely related to the employment structure. A majority of the women (approximately 60 percent) are concentrated in trade in cultural and educational institutions, and in health care, as well as in the textile and clothing industries. Pay in these sectors is relatively low. The better paid positions (e.g. in technical occupations) are chiefly held by men. Women work primarily in the service sectors, in which the pay is lower. A man with more professional training is most often a technician, whereas a woman with advanced professional training is usually a nurse or teacher or she works in trade or administration. In general, the feminized professions are paid less than are the male professions.

The generally lower pay of women cannot, however, be explained wholly by the differing employment structure, as there are differences to the detriment of women within the same profession or sector. An investigation by Lobodzinska (7) of a population of married couples in Warsaw in which both husband and wife work as engineers in the same city planning center has shown that women are hired at a lower level, are promoted less often, and earn less in the same job than do men. On the average, women earn 300 zlotys less than men in the job of senior designer; in the job of designer they earn 150 zlotys less (30 zlotys equal U.S. $1.00). There are even variations of as much as 800 zlotys. These differences are considered by women to be an outrageous injustice to them, especially because the work in planning centers is collective work and each person knows exactly how much another earns. In occupations that require advanced training, these differences are frequently even greater. In the system of fixed pay rates, women are often assigned to the lower limit of the corresponding pay grade.

Unequal Work Positions

The level of pay depends basically on the job (8). Table 3 shows the sex structure in the higher work positions in industry for the years 1964 and 1968. As is obvious, these positions are chiefly occupied by men.

Table 3

Percentage of women in higher work positions
of Polish industry in 1964 and 1968[a]

Position	1964	1968
	%	%
Director	1.9	1.5
Chief engineer, vice-director for technical affairs	2.2	2.3
Vice-director for management	3.6	4.6
Chief mechanic, chief power engineer, chief technician	2.7	4.2
Head of production section	8.2	7.1
Section mechanic, power engineer, technician	9.7	13.9
Senior foreman	1.7	4.0
Foreman	3.9	5.0
Chief bookkeeper	38.2	30.6
Director of finance section	17.5	23.6
Senior financial consultant	37.6	58.2
Financial consultant	50.8	76.9

[a]Source, reference 1, p. 102.

In 1964, approximately half the men with advanced academic training had management positions; in contrast, of 200 women with advanced academic training, only 32 had such a job. Of the men with advanced professional schooling, 45 percent assumed management positions in industry, while less than 10 percent of the women did so. Even in an area so completely feminized as education, scarcely 5.7 percent of women occupied the position of school principal; conversely, one of every five men with higher academic training employed in education occupied such a position (9). Of the 60 women surveyed who worked as engineers in the Warsaw planning centers, only one held a management position; yet one of every four men surveyed held such a position (10).

Psychogenic Differences?

Regarding female labor, the proposition that women are "different" is accepted by political organs, industrial leaders, and the great majority of people, even if they are not always conscious of it. However, neither in Poland nor in other countries have extensive scientific studies been conducted on this point. Consider, for example, the difference in the way women and men approach the choice of occupations, a process from which the division of professions into "male" and "female" results. Normally, this is ascribed to the difference in abilities, propensities, and interests of men and women. Division into "male" and "female" is not, however, based on scientific studies, and men and women are not assigned to a particular job on the basis of such studies. Scientists who have studied this problem in Poland such as Piotrowski, Waluk, Wrochno, and Sokolowska are realizing that the division of professions according to sex is retained above all for traditional reasons, and that, for the same traditional reasons, women are more likely to enter professions for which they are considered suited. The particular suitability of these professions for women is justified by theories according to which women are specially predestined for them, as well as by theories about the "domestic origin" of these professions in which women predominate and which are considered an "extension" of the woman's domestic role.

The division into male and female professions is most clearly evident among workers; as the level of education increases, this distinction decreases. Factors such as training, profession, status in one's profession, age, place of residence, social background, and the profession of one's marital partner are often more important than one's sex. Nevertheless, there is the tendency to emphasize a person's sex and the culturally stipulated "constraints of the elements of sexuality," as Radwilowicz (11), author of a study of the interests of boys and girls in Warsaw schools, has termed it.

Also emphasized is the fact that people's attitudes toward their work are a product of their social milieu, which can be formed and changed. It is likely that biology and motherhood exert a certain influence on the psyche of a woman, but this influence has not yet been researched and is by no means uniform. Possibly there exists a certain specific connection between women's attitude toward their professions and their biology and motherhood; yet there are certainly, perhaps particularly, variable psychic signs that depend on education, values, traditions, cultural ideals, and prevalent ideologies.

Do Women Work Less Well Than Men?

Even in Poland this recurring question cannot be answered as there are no universally valid standards by which to evaluate the work of different groups and categories of work in different professions. The small amount of sound knowledge is valid only for physical work in industrial production. From available material, it follows that the *work productivity of female workers is just as high as that of male workers,* and that a particular branch of industry is not prevented from reaching a high index of productivity because of female workers.

Detailed studies carried out in the fine-mechanical, graphic, photo-optical, and optical factories, as well as in factories of the rubber industry, have yielded no differences whatever between the productivity of male and female workers. A comparison was made between the work productivity of men and women who occupied similar work positions and who were doing similar tasks under technical and organizational conditions that were as nearly equal as possible. Thus, productivity was studied and the work evaluation of men and women was investigated by management. There was no significant difference in the work productivity and suitability by profession of men and women. Nevertheless, in almost all groups studied, the women earned less, and everywhere men occupied positions at the upper limits of the corresponding pay grade, whereas women were at the lower limit or in the middle. Half the foremen and shop heads in the factories surveyed believed that women attained the same work productivity as the men, and more than one of them declared that women were the better workers.

One index of professional productivity frequently used is the number of absentee hours in industry. Studies surveying 37,000 workers in 24 factories in different parts of Poland have shown that the *average number of absent days is lower among women than among men*. Subtracting maternity leave and days off to care for a sick child taken by women and the paid time given to men for military service, the index of days missed per year was 6.8 for women and 8.7 for men (12).

Women without Professional Qualifications

According to data from employment agencies, there were more positions available than there were people looking for work in the years 1966-1970 (13). Yet, in many places, a surplus of women looking for work was recorded. Although it is true that, in the last decade, employment of women accounted for nearly 52 percent of the general increase in employment (a number equal to the number of women offered work), for the past few years the number of women unable to find work also has been growing. In 1955, approximately 17,700 women were registered as seeking work; by 1964, the number had risen to 60,800. For each position designated for women, 2.3 women applied. These were mostly unqualified women workers who, as a rule, have more difficulty finding work than do men of similar qualifications. This is because jobs that require no qualification or training tend to be less suited to women—they are mostly heavy jobs related to great physical strength (e.g. road building, stevedoring, transportation, and similar jobs). These jobs, which are in general prohibited to women by law, are usually fairly well paid; that is one of the reasons for the large differences in the pay level of men and women without professional training. The percentage of men who have not completed primary school education is greater than that of women; nevertheless, it is considerably easier for men to be employed.

In times when economic methods predominated that required quantity rather than quality, employment of people who possessed only limited professional qualifications presented no difficulty. Since the transition to more complicated types of work has taken place, however, the demand for unskilled labor has decreased. This has had a particularly strong effect on the demand for female labor. In areas where labor is lacking, there is an initiative to employ and train unqualified female workers who form the only available reserve. Since about 1972 the number of jobs offered to women (including unqualified women) at both national and local levels has exceeded the number of women looking for jobs. Where there is enough of a labor force, there is less interest in unqualified women. Under certain circumstances, the automatic demand is fulfilled by factors outside the economy, by the initiative of the People's Councils, and by the social organizations. If, however, this is also insufficient, and if places of employment cannot absorb all women, even those with prior training, the creation of additional work positions becomes necessary.

A surplus of female labor during a time when there is also a deficit of male labor can be evidence of an ongoing economic development of a certain area. In the province of Bialystok, which is considered the most underdeveloped province in Poland, women have difficulty finding work (14):

> One could assume that this is simply a specific problem of this agrarian province and is merely evidence of a certain reversal in relation to preceding years when women

were brought in from other areas. The claim that the surplus in the female work force and the deficit in the male work force are both evidence of the progressiveness of this province sounds paradoxical. The fact that women from the villages of this province first seek work outside of farming must still be regarded as a sign of progress for them.

Women without qualifications represent 87 percent of the blue-collar workers employed in the socialized sector of the Polish economy. They work chiefly at such jobs as saleswomen, store managers, maids, messengers, packers, laundresses, and ironers. It is quite characteristic that this range of jobs is not growing. Every restructuring of employment and every so-called "reduction of excess employment" first involves this low-productivity group. If one leans toward rationalization, then immediately the question arises of so-called social employment, i.e. an employment that is motivated rather by social than by economic reasons. This question is primarily raised concerning women without qualifications, but also for wives of alcoholics, widows, unwed mothers, and the like. Also men are often kept on the job for social reasons (for instance, long-time coworkers who are no longer fully capable, poor workers, or drinkers who have to take care of several children). Nevertheless, public opinion believes that the issue of providing employment that is not rationally determined (i.e. employment motivated by goals other than that of economic profit exclusively) is related only to women and the imprecation "problem worker" refers only to females.

Approximately 13 percent of women employed outside agriculture are the sole support of their families. A study made in 1969 has shown that the pay of these women who are the sole support of their families is 15-30 percent below the average pay in each place of employment in question (1). These differences can be attributed to the lower positions and qualifications of single women, for whom the question of training is particularly difficult. Women who are the sole support of their families have priority in using social services, various forms of aid, and loans; they may not be fired. The authors of the 1969 study believe that help for this group of women must include making it easier for these women to educate their children by providing guaranteed places in day-care centers, kindergartens, and summer camps, and by organizing tutoring help for their school-age children. The study showed that 47 percent of the children in question used the day-care centers, 56 percent the kindergartens, and 67 percent the summer camps. The second form of help for this group of women would consist of raising their vocational skills. Women who provide the sole support for their families are usually good workers; they work even better than others because they care more for their jobs. Obtaining vocational training would make it possible for them to advance in their work and thereby to obtain a higher level of pay.

Trends in Employment Policy

There are two trends regarding the employment of women: one toward raising the occupational position of women, and the other toward guaranteeing women conditions that will better enable them to accomplish their domestic duties. The two trends do not contradict each other, but are complementary; however, they emphasize different areas and thus are visible in practice to differing degrees. These differences are most evident among women without any professional qualifications; the higher the level of education, the less evident these differences become.

The first trend is expressed in measures that are intended to raise women's professional qualifications and to improve their work conditions, and to construct day-care centers, kindergartens, and other institutions to help parents care for their children. In addition, there are also trends toward the development of services that make it easier to run a household. The program to raise professional qualifications affects both women without vocational training and also women who must be retrained from occupations in which demand exceeds the supply.

Programs to improve work conditions include: (a) updating and reducing the list of jobs prohibited for women; (b) gradually reducing the number of women who work in the three-shift system; (c) further improving health care for women by constructing a network of consultation clinics; (d) providing protective clothing for working women and adapting machines and implements to the requirements of the female body; and (e) constructing sanitary and hygienic facilities, dressing rooms, washrooms, and breakfast rooms, and improving the lighting and ventilation.

The programs for constructing day-care and educational institutions provide for an increase in the number of places in day-care centers and kindergartens and in the recreation rooms of schools (many children of school age do not have a chance to use the recreation rooms of their schools while their parents are working). An effort is being made to ensure the national economic plan for rapid development of day-care centers, kindergartens, schools, and summer camps, as well as to construct such facilities as recreation rooms and weekday boarding schools. Simultaneously, there must be an attempt to implement the forms of child care, especially for children of preschool age, which best meet the specific needs of the parents (for example, so-called mini-day-care centers and nursery schools for 6-year-old children at the schools).

In the area of services that make household tasks easier, the following programs, among others, are planned: (a) constructing factory cafeterias and food services, and developing expanded programs to earn food in the factories; (b) developing a similar program for the schools, especially the elementary ones; (c) completing a network of grocery stores in the larger settlements and near the large factories, as well as ensuring that these stores are supplied with the items most needed; (d) expanding the availability of precooked or semicooked meals to make work in the kitchen easier; (e) ensuring that the production of constantly needed items, as well as chemical items that make work in the household easier, is developed more quickly; and (f) developing a network of laundries, repair shops, and cleaning services. Much has already been said and written about this in Poland. In actuality, however, the country is not nearly as far along in these areas as are other socialist countries.

The second trend is expressed in measures that tend to bind women more closely to the household. These measures are concentrated somewhat on measures such as increasing the number of half-day positions, promoting at-home work, lengthening maternity leaves, and restricting the level of so-called social employment. The creation of half-day positions for women, especially for married women, has been discussed for years in Poland. In many countries, half-day work for women is quite widespread. In East Germany, 34 percent of the women work half-days in trade, 12 percent in the electronic industry, more than 25 percent in health care services, and more than 36 percent in telecommunications (15). In Poland, however, only 2.5 percent of the women work half-days, and one hears women express the opinion "A half-day position is only half a loaf." A projection of the principles for developing partial employment for women developed in 1971 allows primarily for the necessary elasticity in this form of labor.

In discussing employment policy in the press, the problem of at-home work has again become a public issue. This form of labor has been recognized as a significant element in the development of the economy and in mobilization of the productive reserve. The proposal for at-home work development projects was preceded by numerous studies, consultations, and discussions, which pointed out that at-home work can be applied even in a highly developed country across broad areas with full economic and social benefit. Examples include countries such as Sweden, France, and West Germany. "The development of at-home work accompanied the development of large-scale industrial production in Japan, in many countries of Western Europe, and also in Poland. Aside from expanding the assortment of goods available, at-home work fulfils an important social function: it gives employment to women at home with their children and to invalids" (16). In East Germany the approach to this problem seems somewhat different. A scientific study there about at-home work concluded (17):

> At-home work cannot represent at all the best method for women with domestic responsibilities because this type of work does not, like other kinds of work, create the feeling of a common activity. In addition, there is in this case a *societal isolation* which is felt very deeply and which reinforces any existing physical difficulties. At-home work should primarily be given to: (a) crippled citizens who can work, who possess special knowledge, and who, for reasons of health, are not able to go someplace every day to work, as well as citizens who have to care constantly for family members with severe handicaps; (b) women with several small children or babies whom it is not desirable or possible to accommodate in child-care facilities; (c) women with one baby for whom there is currently no room available in a child-care facility and for whom social reasons justify the acceptance of at-home work.

The introduction of the one-year unpaid "vacation"[1] to care for a child up to the age of two years is also a problem often touched upon in the press. Here are some statements from participants in a discussion on this subject (18):

> In Lodz, studies have shown again that it is only a very small percentage of women who take advantage of this vacation, but also that there are practically no women who take complete advantage of it, that is, use the whole year. They take it only for a short time, usually just for several months [Professor Jerzy Piotrowski, Chairman of the Department for Labor Sociology at the Higher School for Planning and Statistics, Warsaw].
>
> We have been devoting attention for a long time to these vacations, and in the process we have had to overcome opposition from many quarters. At the time all ministers were concerned with what would happen to production. We argued that, if men serve in the military and production does not suffer thereby, women should have the right to have the same conditions for taking care of a very young child. We are not carrying out studies on this subject but we know that, primarily because of the family budget, only approximately 20 percent of the young mothers can afford an unpaid interruption of their work, even if for less than a year. The unions therefore are

---

[1] In January 1972 the one-year vacation was prolonged to three years.

demanding an extension of this leave to three years with financial compensation which could be taken from the sums designated to support children in the day-care centers [Barbara Natorska, Chairwoman of the Board of the Workers Union for the Textile, Clothing and Leather Industry].

It seems to me that the productiveness of such a leave is expressed in a "social" gain, especially for women with low qualifications who, let's say, have three children under 10 or 15 years of age [Doctor Jerzy Holzer, Secretary of the Committee of Demographic Sciences at the Polish Academy of Sciences].

The question of social productiveness has not been completely settled either in this discussion or in practice. One year ago, the rector of the Medical Academy in Warsaw spoke in a similar discussion and noted that the introduction of long and attractive leave could cause hospitals to close because young nurses would take advantage of this leave on a massive scale. Meanwhile, experience has shown that many women still do not completely use the leave as offered in its present form. The birth of a child causes greater expenses for the family; if the mother were to stop working, the income of the family would decrease. There are primarily two groups of women who take advantage of the unpaid leave: women who do not earn much, do most of the housework themselves, and earn additional money by working at odd jobs, and women from families that are already financially secure. The situation, however, is complicated by another factor: for women who do not regard their job as simply a source of money and who want to advance and develop themselves further, a lengthy interruption of their work presents a danger. Even combining this leave with a financial profit could hardly induce the majority of women with higher educational training to interrupt their jobs for a long time. This has been shown by the Hungarian experiment that had different effects at different levels of the population. In Hungary, a three-year leave, combined with a relatively considerable subsidy, has been introduced. Those who take advantage of this form of leave are primarily women with low qualifications.

Education: The Determining Factor of a Woman's Position in the Work Force

Both the experience of everyday life and systematic studies have shown that education is the primary determinant of the position of women in the labor force. Education has a stabilizing effect on professional activity; the higher the level of training and qualification, the weaker the influence of factors making employment difficult for women (such as variations in the economic situation, difficulties in finding work, and domestic duties). Whether a woman is an "unsure" and "burdensome" worker or a sought-after or even indispensable one depends to a significant extent upon her training and qualifications. The higher the qualification and position, the less negative are the consequences of her double load from her duties to her profession and her family. The worker, either male or female, who is interested in his or her work and enjoys it will change or interrupt it less often. The higher the qualification, the more independent and creative the activity, the less the sex of the worker matters, and less emphasis is placed on the differences between men and women in regard to being hired for a particular job. In such cases, the job assumes a continuing high level in the value system; it is an inner need, one of the basic requirements for personal happiness.

Education is the most important of the factors that influence the decision of married women to become employed and that influence their work activities. In Poland, 64 percent of the women with an education of elementary school or less are employed, as are 72 percent who have completed a middle-level professional school, 81 percent who have completed an advanced general education school, 83 percent who have completed an advanced professional school, and 92 percent who have completed their academic education or semiprofessional training (e.g. nursing or teacher training). Only 66 percent of the women with elementary school education, but 95 percent of the women with advanced education, show steady employment with only short interruptions, which are normally related to changing their places of work.

Most women resume work after childbirth. According to a study carried out by Kurzynowski (19) for 1951-1964, two-thirds of the women who take maternity leave return to their jobs. There are, however, noticeable differences among the different groups with varying backgrounds and professions. Training is the deciding factor in this as well; all other factors are only of secondary importance.

More marginal women workers than other categories of women workers give up employment following maternity leave. Table 4 illustrates this point by showing for various occupations the percentage of married women at work six months after the end of their maternity leave.

Giving up one's work, however, is not necessarily proof of lack of interest or of reluctance to work. Often it simply results from the difficulty of coping with work both at home and outside the home and is the consequence of a necessary choice between obligatory and optional duties and responsibilities. Almost all the women questioned by Kurzynowski replied that it had been their wish to continue working after their maternity leave, although many had not been able to do so.

It was also observed in Hungary that training and the type of work have a decisive influence on whether an employed woman interrupts her work or resumes her job after the birth of a child (20). In 1967 a system was introduced there, according to which women can extend their maternity leave up to three years, and according to which they can make claim to a special, rather considerable financial subsidy during this time. The proportion of women who take advantage of this extended leave is, among women with elementary school education, 72 percent; among women with secondary school education, 60 percent; and among women with advanced education, 30 percent. It was also shown that a direct relation exists between the willingness to renounce this subsidy before the end of the legal time period and the level of training: of the women with elementary school education, 15 percent renounced it ahead of time; of those with secondary school education, 25 percent; and of those with advanced education, 46 percent. That leads to the conclusion that women with higher qualifications are more reluctant to accept this form of assistance. All other factors examined—profession, pay, husband's education, age, length of marriage, number of children, type of residence and job, and branch of the economy—were irrelevant or secondary in importance.

The behavior of these women as actually observed does not always agree with the views expressed on the subject of work activity. Numerous studies on the employment of women have been conducted in Poland. In the 1950s, these studies examined female workers only; they were usually asked why they had gone to work. From the

Table 4

Married women again at work six months following
maternity leave, by occupation[a]

Occupation	Percentage Still at Work
	94.7
Doctors and pharmacists	94.2
Nursery school staff	84.9
Engineers and technicians	84.2
Production workers in industry and construction	
Skilled	70.0
Unskilled	49.0
Charwomen	48.0

[a]Source, reference 19, p. 98.

answers of the workers whose educational level was mostly quite low, who were performing jobs for which they had not been trained, who often had many children and earned very little, it was concluded that all women feel less bound to their jobs than men, that liking their work plays less of a role for them, and that they work only because of "economic pressure." It was only in the 1960s that the hiring of other groups of women was studied. A survey carried out by the weekly magazine *Kobieta i Zycie* in 1961 obtained the first statements of well-educated women (1, p.62). Although it was only a press survey, general statements about the people who answered the survey can be made, as these results were confirmed in later systematic studies. The substantial response (2000 answers, although there were more than 60 questions) was evidence of the strong interest of women who were being asked for the first time about their attitudes toward their jobs—teachers, doctors, engineers, and nurses. Personal inclination was given as the first and most important motivation for choosing the job by 84.9 percent of the doctors, 73.6 percent of the teachers, and 67.5 percent of the nurses.

An unskilled or very demanding job is hard to like. The motivations for employment change with the level of training. Training is a factor that makes it easier for women to be accepted in certain positions. Therefore, training determines women's attitudes toward their work and the positions they can attain. The process of change is thus considerably accelerated by training and leads to a reduction of previously existing prejudices and stereotypes that still determine the unequal professional position of women. These stereotypes affect the role and position of women, their abilities, and characteristics, and are rooted both in the women themselves and in their social and professional environment. These stereotypes, however, have no decisive significance; they only inhibit the tempo of the changes and are not able to stop them.

In studies of the motivation and hiring of women, as well as their opinions and attitudes toward their environment, questions such as, "Do you want the work or not?" consumed much thought. The results shed interesting light on the dynamics of the changes that occur with regard to the concept and ideas about the position of women in society. It is remarkable that, generally, people expressed the conviction that women were equal both in society and at work. Such statements have great significance because they give information about the official norms regarded as binding, about the principles of the formerly accepted "catechism," and about the recognized models of social behavior. Between these models and the actual behavior pattern can be more or less strong separating boundaries, depending on the circumstances and the type of behavior being studied. Such material makes no statement about actual behavior, but simply the fact that certain declared models generally exist is evidence of the fact that these are occurrences of great social validity.

The problem of the different attitudes of men and women toward work is of great importance, as it is closely related to the whole concept of future societies. This concept is closely connected with that of the position of women in the world, which in turn is determined principally by their work.

Today, society demands more of women than the fulfilment of their traditional role as women and of their strictly biological role in the continuation of the species. The material and spiritual output of one-half of the human race—of males alone—is no longer enough. Women are needed to work, create, and share with men the responsibility of building the world of tomorrow. Women, who make up the other half of the world's population, constitute a reserve of labor in large part untapped until recently.

Despite the efforts of a decreasing number of supporters of the "traditional system" to prove that employment places too heavy a burden on women, the fact is that the problems arising result from the conflict between the classical image of woman and her actual social functions and responsibilities now. This conflict bears heavily on modern societies, particularly in the industrialized countries.

One's attitude toward work stems from the social structure, which is, itself, subject to change. Scientific research is undermining "static" concepts, even so firmly rooted a concept as that of the immutability of human nature.

REFERENCES

1. Wrochno, K. *Problems of Women's Work,* p. 27. Wydawnictwo Zwiazkowe, Warsaw, 1971 (in Polish).
2. *Statistical Yearbook*, 1927, Tables 22-23, and 1939, Table 28 (in Polish).
3. *Zycie Warszawy* (Warsaw's Life), August 31, 1972.
4. Wrochno, K. *Women in Poland,* pp. 22-27. Interpress, Warsaw, 1969 (in English).
5. Waluk, J. *Remuneration and Work of Women in Poland,* p. 250. Ksiazka i Wiedza, Warsaw, 1965.
6. Waluk, J. On the remuneration of women in Poland. In *Contemporary Woman,* edited by M. Sokolowska, pp. 172-203. Ksiazka i Wiedza, Warsaw, 1966.
7. Lobodzinska, B. Women as engineers. *Problemy Rodziny* 5: 33-39, 1967.
8. Sokolowska, M., and Wrochno, K. The social position of women in the light of statistics. *Studia Socjologiczne* 1(16): 131-159, 1965.
9. Preiss-Zajdowa, A. *Occupation and the Work of Women,* p. 52. Wydawnictwo Zwiazkowe, Warsaw, 1967.
10. Lobodzinska, B. *Urban Marriage,* pp. 161-163. Panstwowe Wydawnictwo Naukowe, Warsaw, 1970.

11. Radwilowicz, R. Interests of male and female pupils. In *Contemporary Woman*, edited by M. Sokolowska, pp. 323-328. Ksiazka i Wiedza, Warsaw, 1966.
12. Stoberski, J. Women and sick leave. *Praca i Zabezpieczenie Spoleczne* 22-26, 1968.
13. Sobczak, L. The problem of hiring women without vocational skills. In *Woman-Work-Household, Proceedings of a Conference*, edited by A. Kloskowska, J. Piotrowski, and K. Wrochno, pp. 22-26. Wydawnictwo Zwiazkowe, Warsaw, 1968.
14. Tryfan, B. Contribution to conference discussion. In *Woman-Work- Household, Proceedings of a Conference*, edited by A. Kloskowska, J. Piotrowski, and K. Wrochno, p. 207. Wydawnictwo Zwiazkowe, Warsaw, 1968.
15. Bankowska, J. Part-time work –Positive and negative aspects. *Zycie Warszawy*, February 21-22, 1971.
16. Tycner, W. Problems of at-home work. *Trybuna Ludu*, February 9, 1971.
17. Renker, U. Heimarbeit. *Wissenschafliche Zeitschrift der Martin-Luther-Universitat Halle-Wittenberg* 2: 155, 157, 1965 (in German).
18. Discussion, *Trybuna Ludu*, March 8, 1971.
19. Kurzynowski, A. *Maternity and Continuity of Work*. Panstwowe Wydawnictwo Ekonomiczne, Warsaw, 1967.
20. Szabady, E. The impact of social factors on the utilization of a prolonged maternity leave in Hungary. *Praca i Zabezpieczenie Spoteczne* 3: 9-15, 1971.

CONTRIBUTORS TO THE VOLUME

ROBIN F. BADGLEY holds cross appointments as a professor of pediatrics and sociology and is chairman of the Department of Behavioural Science, Faculty of Medicine, University of Toronto, Canada. Dr. Badgley has been concerned with issues of public policy relating to the organization of health services, health manpower, and the setting of health priorities. He is coauthor with Dr. Samuel Wolfe of *Doctors' Strike: Medical Care and Conflict in Saskatchewan* (1967) and *The Family Doctor* (1972).

ROBERTO BELMAR is director of the Division of Education of the Department of Social Medicine at Montefiore Hospital and Medical Center and associate professor of community health at the Albert Einstein College of Medicine. Until September 11, 1973 he was associate professor of public health and social medicine at the University of Chile and deputy director of the Fifth Zone (Santiago) of the Chilean National Health Service. Dr. Belmar had his postgraduate training in the Departments of Community Medicine and of Behavioral Sciences of the University of Kentucky (1965-1966) and at the London School of Hygiene and Tropical Medicine (1969-1970). He was awarded a Faculty Fellowship by the Milbank Memorial Fund in 1964, which permitted the development of the program of community medicine in the Faculty of Medicine of the University of Chile. His work has been oriented toward medical education, community medicine, and ambulatory medical care. During the Allende Administration (1970-1973) he actively participated in developing the new model of differentiated levels of ambulatory medical care.

CAROL A. BROWN is assistant professor of urban studies at Queens College, City University of New York, and is a member of the Women's Research Center of Boston. She previously taught at the Heller Graduate School for Social Welfare at Brandeis University. Dr. Brown received her Ph.D. in sociology from Columbia University in 1971. She has written articles on allied health manpower and on divorced mothers, her two main research interests.

BONNIE BULLOUGH is associate professor of community health at the University of California at Los Angeles and associate director of the University Extension Division Pediatric Nurse Practitioner Project. She became a registered nurse in 1947 with a diploma from Salt Lake General Hospital and worked for 15 years in staff nurse positions. Dr. Bullough returned to graduate school at UCLA and earned an M.S. in nursing in 1962. She received her Ph.D. in sociology at UCLA in 1968. Her most recent book is *The Law and the Expanding Nursing Role* (1975). She is also coauthor of *The Emergence of Modern Nursing* (1969), *Poverty, Ethnic Identity and Health Care* (1972), and *Women, Sex and Prostitution* (1975), and is coeditor of two books of readings on the issues in nursing.

KATHLEEN CANNINGS is currently a Ph.D. student in the Department of Urban Studies and Planning at the Massachusetts Institute of Technology. She is doing research on the regional impact of foreign direct investment, particularly in Canada. She has also studied at Brandeis University and Harvard University. Ms. Cannings is a member of the Union for Radical Political Economics.

LEON J. DAVIS is president of District 1199 and its natural union, the National Union of Hospital and Health Care Employees, a Division of RWDSU/AFL-CIO. A former pharmacist, he was one of a small group of drugstore employees who founded the union in 1932. He became the union's first full-time organizer in 1935 and has served as its president for more than 35 years. The union now represents some 100,000 hospital and health care employees in 18 states. In the course of his union activities, he was sentenced to prison twice. He served a 30-day jail sentence in 1962 for refusing to call off a strike at two hospitals in New York City. Again, in 1969, he spent 8 days in jail during the union's historic 113-day hospital strike in Charleston, South Carolina.

BARBARA EHRENREICH is a coauthor of *The American Health Empire: Power, Profits and Politics*; of *Witches, Midwives and Nurses: A History of Women Healers*; and of *Complaints and Disorders: The Sexual Politics of Illness*. She formerly taught in the community health program at the State University of New York, College at Old Westbury, and was a staff member of the Health Policy Advisory Center. She receiver her Ph.D. from Rockefeller University in 1968.

JOHN H. EHRENREICH teaches in the community health and American studies programs at the State University of New York, College at Old Westbury. A former staff member of the Health Policy Advisory Center and of Local 1199, Drug and Hospital Workers Union, he received his Ph.D. from Rockefeller University in 1969. Dr. Ehrenreich is coauthor of *The American Health Empire: Power, Profits and Politics*.

MOE FONER is executive secretary of District 1199 and its national union, the National Union of Hospital and Health Care Employees, a Division of RWDSU/AFL-CIO. He has been with the union since 1952. His responsibilities include such areas as publications and public relations, political action, education, and social and cultural activities. He received the Silver Anvil Award of the American Public Relations Association for his role in publicizing the hospital workers' cause during the union's

154